DASH Diet Cookbook For Beginners

The Ultimate Guide to Managing Blood Pressure Problems, Abundant Low-Sodium Recipes and Mediterranean-Inspired 14-Day Meal Plan.

Gracie Ruiz

Copyright

Disclaimer: The information provided in this book is for educational and informational purposes only. It is not intended as a substitute for professional medical advice, diagnosis, or treatment. Always seek the advice of your physician or other qualified health provider with any questions you may have regarding a medical condition.

Table of Content

Quinoa Salad with Chickpeas and Vegetables
Turkey and Avocado Wrap
Lentil Soup
Chickpea and Spinach Curry
Grilled Salmon Salad
Mediterranean Chickpea Salad
Greek Yogurt Chicken Salad
Roasted Vegetable Quinoa Bowl
Whole Wheat Pasta Primavera
Salmon and Asparagus Foil Packets
Quinoa Stuffed Bell Peppers
Caprese Salad with Whole Wheat Pita
Tuna and White Bean Salad
Eggplant and Tomato Ratatouille
6

DINNER DELIGHT

Baked Salmon with Lemon and Herbs
Grilled Chicken Breast with Roasted Vegetables
Spaghetti Squash Primavera
Teriyaki Tofu Stir-Fry
Baked Cod with Tomato Basil Salsa
Balsamic Glazed Brussels Sprouts with Quinoa
Farro and Roasted Vegetable Bowl
Honey Mustard Glazed Turkey Meatballs
Pomegranate Glazed Chicken
Harvest Chicken Skillet
7

SNACKS & APPETIZERS

Hummus with Veggies
Greek Yogurt Dip
Fresh Fruit Salsa with Whole Grain Chips
Mango Salsa with Cinnamon Tortilla Chips
Cottage Cheese with Pineapple Recipe:
Tuna Lettuce Wraps Recipe:

1

INTRODUCTION

The **DASH** (Dietary Approaches to Stop Hypertension) Diet is a dietary plan designed to prevent and manage hypertension (high blood pressure). Here's an overview:

Key Principles:

Emphasis on Fruits and Vegetables: Promotes a high intake of fruits and vegetables, rich in vitamins, minerals, and antioxidants.

Whole Grains: Encourages the consumption of whole grains, such as brown rice, whole wheat, and oats, for fiber and nutrients.

Lean Proteins: Recommends lean protein sources, like poultry, fish, beans, and nuts, while minimizing red meat consumption.

Dairy: Includes low fat or fat free dairy products for calcium and other essential nutrients.

Limited Sodium: Emphasizes reducing sodium (salt) intake to help manage blood pressure. This involves minimizing processed foods and using herbs and spices for flavor.

Moderate Alcohol: Suggests moderate alcohol consumption, if at all, with a focus on healthier options like red wine.

Portion Control: Encourages mindful eating and portion control to maintain a healthy weight.

Implementation:

- **Meal Planning:** Involves creating well balanced meals with a variety of food groups.

- **Regular Exercise:** Often recommended in conjunction with the diet for overall health benefits.

The DASH Diet is recognized for its positive impact on heart health and is often recommended by healthcare professionals as part of a comprehensive approach to managing blood pressure and promoting overall wellbeing.

Benefits of Following the DASH Diet

Following the DASH (Dietary Approaches to Stop Hypertension) Diet offers several health benefits:

1. **Blood Pressure Management:** The primary goal of the DASH Diet is to lower and manage blood pressure effectively. It has been shown to significantly reduce both systolic and diastolic blood pressure.

2. **Heart Health:** The DASH Diet promotes heart health by emphasizing nutrient dense foods like fruits, vegetables, whole grains, and lean proteins. This helps reduce the risk of cardiovascular diseases.

3. **Weight Management:** The focus on whole foods and portion control can contribute to weight maintenance or weight loss, promoting a healthy body weight.

4. **Reduced Risk of Chronic Diseases:** Following the DASH Diet is associated with a lower risk of chronic conditions such as heart disease, stroke, and certain types of cancer.

5. **Improved Cholesterol Levels:** The diet's emphasis on whole grains, fruits, and vegetables can positively impact cholesterol levels, promoting a healthier lipid profile.

6. **Better Blood Sugar Control:** The DASH Diet's balanced approach may help improve insulin sensitivity and contribute to better blood sugar control, reducing the risk of type 2 diabetes.

7. **NutrientRich Diet:** By encouraging the consumption of a variety of nutrient rich foods, the DASH Diet provides essential vitamins, minerals, and antioxidants, supporting overall wellbeing.

8. **Reduced Sodium Intake:** The DASH Diet's emphasis on limiting sodium intake helps manage blood pressure and reduces the risk of related health issues.

9. **Balanced Nutrition:** The diet encourages a well balanced intake of carbohydrates, proteins, and fats, ensuring a comprehensive and sustainable approach to nutrition.

10. **Lifestyle Integration:** The DASH Diet is often recommended alongside other healthy lifestyle practices, such as regular physical activity, to maximize its benefits.

Tips for success

Achieving success with the DASH (Dietary Approaches to Stop Hypertension) Diet involves adopting a sustainable and mindful approach to your eating habits. Here are some tips for success:

1. **Gradual Changes:** Start by making gradual changes to your diet. This can make the transition more manageable and increase the likelihood of long term success.

2. **Meal Planning:** Plan your meals in advance to ensure they align with DASH Diet principles. This helps you make healthier choices and reduces the temptation of opting for less nutritious options.

3. **Emphasize Whole Foods:** Prioritize whole, unprocessed foods such as fruits, vegetables, whole grains, lean proteins, and low fat dairy. These foods provide essential nutrients without added sugars and excessive salt.

4. **Mindful Eating:** Practice mindful eating by paying attention to your hunger and fullness cues. Avoid distractions while eating, savor your food, and listen to your body's signals.

5. **Portion Control:** Be mindful of portion sizes to avoid overeating. Use smaller plates, bowls, and utensils to help control portions.

6. **Read Labels:** Learn to read food labels to identify hidden sources of sodium and make informed choices. Opt for products with lower sodium content and minimal additives

7. **Healthy Cooking Methods:** Choose healthier cooking methods such as grilling, baking, steaming, or sautéing instead of frying. These methods retain more nutrients and often require less added fat.

8. **Stay Hydrated:** Drink plenty of water throughout the day. Hydration is essential for overall health and can also help with weight management.

9. **Limit Processed Foods:** Reduce your intake of processed and packaged foods, as they often contain high levels of sodium, added sugars, and unhealthy fats.

10. **Include Variety:** Keep your meals interesting by incorporating a variety of fruits, vegetables, and proteins. Experiment with different herbs and spices to add flavor without relying on salt.

11. **Regular Physical Activity:** Combine the DASH Diet with regular physical activity. Exercise is crucial for overall health and complements the diet in managing blood pressure and maintaining a healthy weight.

12. **Seek Support:** Share your DASH Diet journey with friends, family, or support groups. Having a support system can provide encouragement and motivation

13. **Celebrate Progress:** Acknowledge and celebrate your achievements along the way. Whether it's reaching a weight loss goal or consistently making healthier food choices, recognizing your progress can help you stay motivated.

2

UNDERSTANDING THE DASH DIET PRINCIPLES

Key Components of the DASH Diet

The key components of the DASH (Dietary Approaches to Stop Hypertension) Diet include:

1. High Consumption of Fruits and Vegetables:
2. Emphasizes a variety of colorful fruits and vegetables rich in vitamins, minerals, and antioxidants.
3. Aim for multiple servings daily to promote heart health.

2. Whole Grains:

- Recommends whole grains such as brown rice, quinoa, oats, and whole wheat.
- Provides fiber and essential nutrients while supporting overall wellbeing.

3. Lean Proteins:

- Encourages lean protein sources, including poultry, fish, beans, lentils, and nuts.
- Limits red meat consumption, opting for healthier protein options.

4. LowFat or FatFree Dairy:

- Includes low fat or fat free dairy products like milk, yogurt, and cheese.

- Provides calcium and other nutrients without excess saturated fats.

5. Limited Sodium (Salt) Intake:

- Recommends reducing sodium intake to help manage blood pressure.
- Involves minimizing the use of salt in cooking and being mindful of sodium content in processed foods.

6. Moderate Intake of Nuts, Seeds, and Legumes:

- Incorporates nuts, seeds, and legumes for additional protein, fiber, and healthy fats.
- Contributes to satiety and overall nutritional balance.

7. Limited Sweets and Added Sugars:

- Advises limiting the consumption of sweets and added sugars.
- Encourages natural sweetness from fruits and minimizes reliance on sugary snacks.

8. Moderate Alcohol Consumption:

- Suggests moderate alcohol intake, if at all, with a focus on healthier options like red wine.
- Moderation is key to avoiding potential negative health effects.

9. Portion Control:

- Emphasizes portion control to manage calorie intake and support weight management.
- Uses smaller plates and bowls to help control portion sizes.

10. Balanced Nutrient Profile:

- Promotes a balanced intake of carbohydrates, proteins, and healthy fats.
- Ensures a well rounded diet that meets nutritional needs.

11. Overall HeartHealthy Lifestyle:

Recommends combining the DASH Diet with other heart healthy practices, such as regular physical activity and maintaining a healthy weight.

By incorporating these key components, the DASH Diet aims to create a well balanced and nutrient dense eating plan that supports cardiovascular health and helps manage blood pressure.

Sodium Guidelines

The sodium guidelines recommended by the DASH (Dietary Approaches to Stop Hypertension) Diet are designed to help manage blood pressure. Here are the general sodium guidelines:

1. Total Sodium Intake:

- Aim to consume no more than 2,300 milligrams of sodium per day. This is the standard recommendation for most adults.

2. Lower Sodium Intake for Specific Groups:

- If you are at higher risk of hypertension, are older than 50, or have certain health conditions, including diabetes or kidney disease, the recommended daily sodium intake may be even lower—typically around 1,500 milligrams.

3. Gradual Reduction:

- If you currently consume a higher amount of sodium, gradually reduce your intake to allow your taste buds to adjust. Sudden drastic changes may make the adjustment more challenging.

4. Be Mindful of Processed Foods:

- The majority of sodium in the average diet comes from processed and packaged foods. Be vigilant about reading food labels to identify hidden sources of sodium.

5. Use Herbs and Spices for Flavor:

- Reduce reliance on salt for flavoring and experiment with herbs, spices, and other seasonings to enhance the taste of your meals.

6. Limit HighSodium Condiments:

- Be cautious with high sodium condiments such as soy sauce, teriyaki sauce, and certain salad dressings. Opt for reduced sodium versions or use them sparingly.

7. Cook at Home:

- Cooking meals at home allows you to have better control over the ingredients and sodium content. Use fresh, whole ingredients and minimize the use of processed items.

8. Choose Fresh and Frozen Produce:

- Fresh and frozen fruits and vegetables are generally lower in sodium compared to canned varieties. If using canned options, look for those labeled "no added salt" or "low sodium."

9. Drink Plenty of Water:

- Staying well hydrated with water can help flush excess sodium from your system.

10. **Consult with Healthcare Professionals:**

- Individuals with specific health conditions or those on restricted diets should consult with healthcare professionals to determine the appropriate sodium intake for their situation.

Portion Control

Portion control is a key aspect of the DASH (Dietary Approaches to Stop Hypertension) Diet, helping individuals manage their calorie intake and support weight management. Here are some tips for effective portion control:

1. **Use Smaller Plates and Bowls:**

- Opt for smaller dishware to naturally reduce portion sizes. This can help prevent overeating by creating the illusion of a fuller plate.

2. **Divide Your Plate:**

- **Follow the DASH Diet's plate division:** fill half your plate with vegetables, one quarter with lean protein, and one quarter with whole grains. This promotes a balanced and nutritious meal.

3. **Be Mindful of Calories:**

- Pay attention to portion sizes in relation to your daily caloric needs. Consuming appropriate portions helps maintain a healthy weight.

4. **Avoid Eating Straight from the Package:**

- Serve yourself a proper portion rather than eating directly from containers or bags. This makes it easier to keep track of how much you're consuming.

5. **Listen to Hunger Cues:**

- Pay attention to your body's signals of hunger and fullness. Eat slowly and stop when you feel satisfied rather than overly full.

6. **Practice Moderation:**

- Enjoy treats and indulgent foods in moderation. You don't have to eliminate them entirely, but be mindful of portion sizes.

7. **Use Measuring Tools:**

- Initially, use measuring cups or a food scale to gauge proper portion sizes. This can help you develop a better understanding of appropriate serving sizes.

8. **Plan Snacks:**

- Prepare healthy snacks in advance and portion them into individual servings. This helps avoid mindless snacking and promotes better control over calorie intake.

9. **Share Meals at Restaurants:**

- When dining out, consider sharing entrees or ordering smaller portions. Many restaurant servings are larger than necessary.

10. **Avoid Distractions:**

- Eat without distractions, such as watching TV or using electronic devices. This allows you to focus on your meal and recognize when you're satisfied.

11. Don't Skip Meals:

- Regular meals and snacks can help prevent excessive hunger, making it easier to control portions and resist overeating.

12. Stay Hydrated:

- Drink water before meals to help curb appetite and avoid overeating. Sometimes, feelings of thirst can be mistaken for hunger.

3

GETTING STARTED

Kitchen Essentials for the DASH Diet

Having the right kitchen essentials can make it easier to follow the DASH (Dietary Approaches to Stop Hypertension) Diet and prepare healthy meals. Here's a list of kitchen essentials for the DASH Diet:

1. **Measuring Cups and Spoons:**

   - Essential for accurately portioning ingredients and controlling serving sizes.

2. **Food Scale:**

   - Useful for measuring precise amounts of ingredients, especially when first starting to practice portion control.

3. **Cutting Boards:**

   - Have separate cutting boards for fruits, vegetables, and meats to prevent cross contamination.

4. **Sharp Knives:**

   - A set of good quality knives makes chopping and preparing fruits and vegetables more efficient.

5. **Blender or Food Processor:**

- Ideal for making smoothies, purees, and homemade sauces using fresh and whole ingredients.

6. Steamer Basket:

- Makes it easy to steam vegetables while preserving their nutrients.

7. NonStick Pans:

- Require less oil for cooking and are easier to clean.

8. Baking Sheets and Pans:

- Useful for roasting vegetables, lean proteins, and preparing healthy baked goods.

9. Ovenproof Casserole Dish:

- Perfect for creating one dish meals that combine a variety of DASHfriendly ingredients.

10. Grill or Grill Pan:

- Ideal for grilling lean proteins and vegetables, adding a flavorful touch without excess fat.

11. Mixing Bowls:

- Multiple sizes for mixing, tossing salads, or preparing various components of a meal.

12. Herbs and Spices:

- Build a collection of herbs and spices to add flavor to your meals without relying on excessive salt.

13. **Vegetable Peeler:**

- Makes it easy to peel vegetables for salads or cooking.

14. **Storage Containers:**

- Invest in containers for leftovers, making it convenient to store and reheat meals.

15. **Salad Spinner:**

- Helps rinse and dry fresh produce efficiently for salads and other dishes.

16. **Citrus Juicer:**

- Useful for extracting fresh juice from lemons, limes, and oranges to add natural flavor.

17. **NonStick Cooking Spray:**

- A healthier alternative to oils for greasing pans or adding a light coating to vegetables.

18. **Food Storage Bags and Wraps:**

- Use environmentally friendly options for storing and transporting food.

19. **Cutting Shears:**

- Handy for quickly chopping herbs or cutting through small pieces of meat.

20. **Spatulas and Ladles:**

- Essential for stirring, flipping, and serving dishes.

Meal Planning Basics

Meal planning is a fundamental aspect of the DASH (Dietary Approaches to Stop Hypertension) Diet, helping you prepare balanced and nutritious meals. Here are some meal planning basics to get you started:

1. **Set Goals:**

- Define your nutritional goals, whether it's managing blood pressure, weight loss, or overall heart health. Tailor your meal plan to meet these objectives.

2. **Understand DASH Principles:**

- Familiarize yourself with the key components of the DASH Diet, emphasizing fruits, vegetables, whole grains, lean proteins, and limited sodium.

3. **Create a Weekly Schedule:**

- Plan your meals for the week, including breakfast, lunch, dinner, and snacks. Having a schedule helps you stay organized and make healthier choices.

4. **Batch Cooking:**

- Consider batch cooking certain items, such as grains, proteins, or sauces, to save time during the week. This can streamline meal preparation.

5. **Incorporate Variety:**

- Include a variety of foods in your meals to ensure you get a broad range of nutrients. Rotate protein sources, try different vegetables, and experiment with whole grains.

6. **Plan for Leftovers:**

- Plan meals that can yield leftovers for the next day. This reduces cooking time and helps prevent the temptation of less healthy food choices.

7. **Balance Your Plate:**

- Follow the DASH Diet plate division: fill half your plate with vegetables, one quarter with lean protein, and one quarter with whole grains.

8. **Snack Smart:**

- Plan for nutritious snacks between meals to keep your energy levels stable. Include options like fresh fruit, vegetables with hummus, or Greek yogurt.

9. **Consider Meal Prep Containers:**

- Invest in reusable containers to portion out and store your meals. This makes it easy to grab a healthy option when you're on the go.

10. **Check Your Pantry:**

- Take stock of pantry staples and incorporate them into your meal planning. This can help reduce food waste and save money.

11. **Experiment with New Recipes:**

* Keep things interesting by trying new recipes. This prevents boredom and encourages a diverse, nutrient rich diet.

12. **Mindful Grocery Shopping:**

* Stick to your grocery list and choose whole, fresh foods. Read labels to check for sodium content and opt for healthier alternatives.

13. **Prep Ingredients:**

* Wash, chop, and prep ingredients in advance. Having ingredients ready can make cooking during busy weekdays more manageable.

14. **Consider Dietary Preferences and Restrictions:**

* Tailor your meal plan to accommodate any dietary preferences, restrictions, or allergies.

15. **Review and Adjust:**

* Regularly review your meal plan to see what worked well and what can be improved. Adjust your plan based on your preferences and lifestyle.

4

BREAK FAST RECIPE

Whole Grain Breakfast Bowl

Serving: 1 serving   **Total time:** 10 minutes (preparation and assembly)

Ingredients:

- $^1/_2$ cup cooked quinoa or steel cut oats
- $^1/_2$ cup plain Greek yogurt
- $^1/_2$ cup fresh mixed berries (e.g., blueberries, strawberries, raspberries)
- 1 tablespoon honey or maple syrup
- 1 tablespoon chia seeds
- 1 tablespoon chopped nuts (e.g., almonds, walnuts)
- $^1/_2$ banana, sliced
- A sprinkle of cinnamon

Instructions:

1. Follow the directions on the package to cook the steel-cut oats or quinoa. Let them cool somewhat before assembling your bowl together.

2. Place the cooked whole grains in the bottom of a bowl.

3. Make a layer on top of the whole grains by spooning the plain Greek yogurt over them.

4. Fill the bowl with a generous portion of fresh mixed berries. Berries are high in antioxidants and naturally delicious.

5. For extra sweetness, drizzle some honey or maple syrup over the yogurt and berries. Adjust the quantity to your personal taste.

6. Sprinkle chia seeds over the bowl. Chia seeds are rich in fiber and healthy omega-3 fatty acids.

7. Add chopped nuts, such as walnuts or almonds, to the top for extra protein and crunch.

8. Arrange banana slices in the bowl for extra sweetness and a creamy texture.

9. Finish off with a sprinkle of cinnamon, which adds warmth and flavor without additional calories.

Enjoy your nutritious and tasty wholegrain breakfast bowl!

Veggie Omelette

Serving: 1 **Preparation Time:** Approximately 10 minutes **Cooking Time:** 57 minutes (optional, as cooking times may vary) **Total Time:** 1hr 7 minutes

---

Ingredients:

- 2 large eggs
- Salt and pepper to taste

- 1 tablespoon olive oil or cooking spray
- $^1/_4$ cup diced bell peppers (any color)
- $^1/_4$ cup diced tomatoes
- $^1/_4$ cup diced onions
- $^1/_4$ cup chopped spinach or kale
- $^1/_4$ cup shredded cheese (optional)
- Fresh herbs (e.g., parsley, chives) for garnish (optional)
- Salsa or hot sauce for serving (optional)

Instructions:

1. Dice bell peppers, tomatoes, and onions. Chop spinach or kale. Set aside.
2. In a bowl, whisk the eggs until well combined. Season with salt and pepper to taste.
3. Heat olive oil in a nonstick skillet over medium heat. Add diced bell peppers, tomatoes, onions, and chopped spinach or kale. Sauté until vegetables are tender, about 34 minutes.
4. Pour the whisked eggs over the sautéed vegetables, ensuring an even distribution.
5. Allow the eggs to set around the edges. Gently lift the edges with a spatula, tilting the pan to let the uncooked eggs flow to the edges. Cook until the bottom is set but the top is still slightly runny.
6. If using cheese, sprinkle it over one-half of the omelet.
7. Carefully fold the omelet in half using the spatula. Slide it onto a plate.
8. Garnish with fresh herbs if desired. Serve your veggie omelet hot with salsa or hot sauce on the side, if you like.

Enjoy your nutritious and tasty veggie omelet!

Banana Walnut Muffins (Whole Wheat)

Serving: 12 muffins

Preparation Time: Approximately 15 minutes
Baking Time: 20 minutes
Total Time: Approximately 35 minutes

Ingredients:

- 2 ripe bananas, mashed
- $^1/_3$ cup melted coconut oil or unsalted butter
- $^1/_2$ cup honey or maple syrup
- 1 teaspoon vanilla extract
- 2 large eggs
- 1 cup whole wheat flour
- 1 teaspoon baking soda
- $^1/_2$ teaspoon salt
- $^1/_2$ teaspoon ground cinnamon
- $^1/_2$ cup chopped walnuts
- $^1/_4$ cup plain Greek yogurt for added moisture (optional)

Instructions:

1. Preheat your oven to 350°F (175°C). Line a muffin tin with paper liners or grease each cup.
2. In a large mixing bowl, mash the ripe bananas with a fork or potato masher.
3. Add melted coconut oil or butter, honey or maple syrup, vanilla extract, and eggs to the mashed bananas. Mix well until combined.
4. In a separate bowl, whisk together whole wheat flour, baking soda, salt, and ground cinnamon.

5. Gradually add the dry ingredients to the wet ingredients, stirring until just combined. Avoid overmixing to keep the muffins tender.
6. Gently fold in the chopped walnuts. If desired, add plain Greek yogurt for added moisture.
7. Spoon the batter into the prepared muffin cups, filling each about two thirds full.
8. Bake in the preheated oven for 20 minutes or until a toothpick inserted into the center of a muffin comes out clean.
9. Allow the muffins to cool in the tin for a few minutes before transferring them to a wire rack to cool completely.

Oatmeal with Berries

Serving: 1 **Preparation Time**: 5 minutes **Cooking Time:** 5 minutes (microwave) or 15 minutes (stovetop) **Total Time:** 10 minutes (microwave) or 20 minutes (stovetop)

Ingredients:

- $^1/_2$ cup rolled oats
- 1 cup milk (dairy or plant based)
- $^1/_2$ cup mixed berries (blueberries, strawberries, raspberries)
- 1 tablespoon honey or maple syrup
- toppings (optional): sliced almonds, chia seeds

Instructions:

1. In a saucepan or microwave safe bowl, combine rolled oats and milk.

2. If using a stovetop, bring the mixture to a simmer over medium heat, stirring occasionally. If using a microwave, heat on high for 23 minutes, pausing to stir halfway.
3. Once the oats are cooked, remove from heat or microwave.
4. Stir in the mixed berries and sweeten with honey or maple syrup.
5. **Optional:** Top with sliced almonds or chia seeds for added texture and nutrition.
6. Allow the oatmeal to cool slightly before serving.

Greek Yogurt Parfait

Serving: 1 **Preparation Time:** 5 minutes **Assembly Time:** 2 minutes **Total Time:** 7 minutes

Ingredients:

- 1 cup Greek yogurt
- $^1/_2$ cup granola
- $^1/_2$ cup mixed berries (strawberries, blueberries, raspberries)
- 1 tablespoon honey
- Optional: sliced bananas, chopped nuts

Instructions:

1. In a glass or bowl, start by layering half of the Greek yogurt at the bottom.
2. Add a layer of granola on top of the yogurt.
3. Place a layer of mixed berries on the granola.
4. Drizzle honey over the berries.
5. Repeat the layers with the remaining Greek yogurt, granola, and berries.

6. Optional: Garnish with sliced bananas or chopped nuts for extra flavor and texture.
7. Serve immediately and enjoy your delightful Greek Yogurt Parfait!

Smoothie Bowl

Serving: 1   **Preparation Time:** 5 minutes   **Total Time:** 5 minutes

Ingredients:

- 1 frozen banana, sliced
- $^1/_2$ cup frozen mixed berries (strawberries, blueberries, raspberries)
- $^1/_2$ cup Greek yogurt
- $^1/_4$ cup almond milk (or any preferred milk)
- Toppings: granola, sliced fruits (kiwi, berries), chia seeds, shredded coconut.

Instructions:

1. In a blender, combine the frozen banana slices, frozen mixed berries, Greek yogurt, and almond milk.
2. Blend until smooth and creamy, adding more liquid if needed to achieve the desired consistency.
3. Pour the smoothie into a bowl.
4. Arrange toppings on the smoothie surface try granola, sliced fruits, chia seeds, and shredded coconut for variety.
5. Serve immediately and enjoy your vibrant and nutritious smoothie bowl!

Whole Wheat Pancakes

Serving: 8 pancakes **Preparation Time:** 10 minutes **Cooking Time:** 10 minutes **Total Time:** 20 minutes

---

Ingredients:

- 1 cup whole wheat flour
- 1 tablespoon sugar
- 1 teaspoon baking powder
- 1/2 teaspoon baking soda
- 1/4 teaspoon salt
- 1 cup buttermilk (or mix 1 cup milk with 1 tablespoon vinegar)
- 1 large egg
- 2 tablespoons melted butter or oil
- Cooking spray or additional butter for the pan

Instructions:

1. In a large bowl, whisk together the whole wheat flour, sugar, baking powder, baking soda, and salt.
2. In another bowl, whisk together the buttermilk, egg, and melted butter or oil.
3. Pour the wet ingredients into the dry ingredients and stir until just combined. Don't overmix; a few lumps are okay.
4. Heat a griddle or non-stick skillet over medium heat. Lightly coat with cooking spray or butter.
5. Pour 1/4 cup portions of batter onto the griddle for each pancake. Cook until bubbles form on the surface, then flip and cook until golden brown on the other side.
6. Repeat until all the batter is used.

Avocado Toast

Serving: 2 slices of toast **Preparation Time:** 5 minutes **Cooking Time:** 5 minutes **Total Time:** 10 minutes

---

Ingredients:

- 2 slices whole grain bread
- 1 ripe avocado
- Salt and pepper to taste
- **Optional toppings:** red pepper flakes, cherry tomatoes, poached egg, or a sprinkle of feta cheese

Instructions:

1. Toast the whole grain bread slices to your liking.
2. While the bread is toasting, halve the ripe avocado and remove the pit. Scoop the avocado into a bowl.
3. Mash the avocado with a fork and add a pinch of salt and pepper to taste.
4. Once the bread is toasted, spread the mashed avocado evenly on each slice.
5. Add any optional toppings of your choice, such as red pepper flakes, sliced cherry tomatoes, a poached egg, or a sprinkle of feta cheese.
6. Serve immediately and enjoy your delicious and nutrient-packed avocado toast!

Avocado toast is not only quick and easy to make but also a versatile dish that you can customize with your favorite toppings.

Quinoa Breakfast Bowl

Serving: 2 bowls **Preparation Time:** 5 minutes **Cooking Time:** 15 minutes **Total Time:** 20 minutes

---

Ingredients:

- 1 cup quinoa, rinsed
- 2 cups almond milk (or any milk of your choice)
- 1 teaspoon vanilla extract
- 1 tablespoon honey or maple syrup
- Fresh fruits (e.g., berries, sliced banana)
- Nuts and seeds (e.g., almonds, chia seeds)
- Greek yogurt or plant-based yogurt
- Optional: a dash of cinnamon or nutmeg

Instructions:

1. In a medium saucepan, combine the quinoa, almond milk, and vanilla extract.
2. Bring the mixture to a boil, then reduce the heat to low, cover, and simmer for about 15 minutes, or until the quinoa is cooked and most of the liquid is absorbed.
3. Remove from heat and let it sit, covered, for a few minutes. Fluff the quinoa with a fork.
4. Stir in honey or maple syrup for sweetness.
5. Divide the cooked quinoa into bowls.
6. Top each bowl with fresh fruits, nuts, seeds, and a dollop of Greek yogurt or plant-based yogurt.
7. Optionally, sprinkle with a dash of cinnamon or nutmeg for added flavor.
8. Serve warm and enjoy your wholesome Quinoa Breakfast Bowl!

Cottage Cheese and Pineapple

Serving: 1 **Preparation Time:** 5 minutes

Ingredients:

- 1 cup cottage cheese
- 1 cup fresh pineapple chunks

Instructions:

1. In a bowl, spoon out the cottage cheese.
2. Add fresh pineapple chunks on top.

Sweet Potato Hash

Serving: 2 **Preparation Time:** 10 minutes **Cooking Time:** 20 minutes
Total Time: 30 minutes

Ingredients:

- 2 medium sweet potatoes, peeled and diced
- 1 red bell pepper, diced
- 1 small red onion, diced
- 2 tablespoons olive oil
- 1 teaspoon smoked paprika
- $1/2$ teaspoon garlic powder
- Salt and pepper to taste

- **Optional toppings:** poached or fried eggs, avocado slices, fresh herbs

Instructions:

1. Heat olive oil in a large skillet over medium heat.
2. Add diced sweet potatoes to the skillet and cook for about 10 minutes, stirring occasionally, until they start to soften.
3. Add diced red bell pepper and red onion to the skillet. Continue to cook for another 8-10 minutes, or until all vegetables are tender and slightly crispy.
4. Sprinkle smoked paprika, garlic powder, salt, and pepper over the hash. Stir to combine and cook for an additional 2-3 minutes.
5. **Optional:** In a separate pan, prepare poached or fried eggs.
6. Serve the sweet potato hash on plates, topped with poached or fried eggs, avocado slices, and fresh herbs if desired.

Chia Seed Pudding

Serving: 2 **Preparation Time:** 5 minutes (plus chilling time)

Ingredients:

- $^1/_4$ cup chia seeds
- 1 cup almond milk (or any milk of your choice)
- 1 tablespoon honey or maple syrup
- $^1/_2$ teaspoon vanilla extract
- Fresh fruits for topping (e.g., berries, sliced banana)
- Nuts and seeds for topping (e.g., sliced almonds, chia seeds)

Instructions:

1. In a bowl, whisk together chia seeds, almond milk, honey or maple syrup, and vanilla extract.
2. Whisk the mixture well to ensure the chia seeds are evenly distributed.
3. Cover the bowl and refrigerate for at least 2 hours or overnight. Stir occasionally during the first 30 minutes to prevent clumping.
4. After the chia pudding has set, give it a good stir.
5. Divide the chia seed pudding into serving bowls or jars.
6. Top with fresh fruits and your choice of nuts and seeds.
7. Optionally, drizzle with additional honey or maple syrup if desired.

Fruit Salad

Serving: 2 **Preparation Time:** 10 minutes

Ingredients:

- 1 cup strawberries, hulled and sliced
- 1 cup pineapple chunks
- 1 cup grapes, halved
- 1 kiwi, peeled and sliced
- 1 banana, sliced
- Fresh mint leaves for garnish (optional)
- Honey or lime juice for drizzling (optional)

Instructions:

1. In a large bowl, combine the strawberries, pineapple chunks, grapes, kiwi slices, and banana slices.

2. Gently toss the fruits together until well mixed.
3. **Optional:** Drizzle honey or lime juice over the fruit salad for added sweetness or a citrusy kick.
4. Garnish with fresh mint leaves for a burst of flavor (optional).
5. Serve immediately, or refrigerate for a short time if you prefer a chilled fruit salad.

Muesli with Almond Milk

Serving: 1 **Preparation Time:** 5 minutes

Ingredients:

- $^1/_2$ cup muesli (store-bought or homemade)
- 1 cup almond milk
- Fresh fruits (e.g., berries, sliced banana)
- Nuts and seeds (e.g., almonds, chia seeds)
- Optional: a drizzle of honey or maple syrup

Instructions:

1. In a bowl, combine the muesli and almond milk.
2. Stir well to ensure the muesli is evenly soaked in the almond milk.
3. Let it sit for a couple of minutes to allow the muesli to absorb the almond milk.
4. Top with fresh fruits, nuts, and seeds of your choice.
5. Optionally, drizzle with honey or maple syrup for added sweetness.
6. Give it a final gentle stir before enjoying.

Spinach and Feta Frittata

Serving: 4 **Preparation Time:** 10 minutes **Cooking Time:** 15 minutes
Total Time: 25 minutes

Ingredients:

- 6 large eggs
- 1 cup fresh spinach, chopped
- $^1/_2$ cup feta cheese, crumbled
- $^1/_2$ cup cherry tomatoes, halved
- $^1/_4$ cup red onion, finely chopped
- 2 tablespoons olive oil
- Salt and pepper to taste
- Fresh herbs for garnish (e.g., parsley or dill)

Instructions:

1. Preheat the oven to 375°F (190°C).
2. In a bowl, whisk the eggs until well beaten. Season with salt and pepper.
3. In an oven-safe skillet, heat olive oil over medium heat.
4. Add chopped spinach, red onion, and cherry tomatoes to the skillet. Cook for 2-3 minutes until the vegetables are slightly softened.
5. Pour the whisked eggs over the vegetables in the skillet. Allow the eggs to set around the edges.
6. Sprinkle crumbled feta cheese evenly over the eggs.
7. Transfer the skillet to the preheated oven and bake for about 10-12 minutes or until the frittata is set in the center and lightly golden on top.
8. Remove from the oven, let it cool for a few minutes, then slice into wedges.
9. Garnish with fresh herbs before serving.

Peanut Butter Banana Wrap

Serving: 1 wrap **Preparation Time:** 5 minutes

Ingredients:

- 1 whole wheat wrap or tortilla
- 2 tablespoons peanut butter
- 1 banana, sliced
- **Optional:** a drizzle of honey or a sprinkle of cinnamon

Instructions:

1. Lay the whole wheat wrap or tortilla on a flat surface.
2. Spread the peanut butter evenly over the surface of the wrap.
3. Place banana slices in a row along one edge of the wrap.
4. **Optional:** Drizzle honey or sprinkle cinnamon over the banana slices for added sweetness.
5. Roll the wrap tightly from the banana-covered edge, creating a snug wrap.
6. Slice the wrap in half if desired, and serve.

5

LUNCH RECIPES/IDEAS

Quinoa Salad with Chickpeas and Vegetables

Serving: 4 servings **Preparation Time**: 15 minutes **Cooking Time:** 15 minutes (for quinoa) **Total Time:** 30 minutes

---

Ingredients:

- 1 cup quinoa, rinsed
- 2 cups water or vegetable broth (for cooking quinoa)
- 1 can (15 oz) chickpeas, drained and rinsed
- 1 cup cherry tomatoes, halved
- 1 cucumber, diced
- 1 bell pepper (any color), diced
- $^1/_4$ cup red onion, finely chopped
- $^1/_4$ cup feta cheese, crumbled
- $^1/_4$ cup fresh parsley, chopped

For the Dressing:

- 3 tablespoons olive oil
- 2 tablespoons lemon juice
- 1 teaspoon Dijon mustard
- 1 clove garlic, minced
- Salt and pepper to taste

Instructions:

1. Rinse quinoa under cold water. In a saucepan, combine quinoa and water or vegetable broth. Bring to a boil, then reduce heat, cover, and simmer for 15 minutes or until quinoa is cooked and water is absorbed.
2. In a large bowl, combine cooked quinoa, chickpeas, cherry tomatoes, cucumber, bell pepper, red onion, feta cheese, and fresh parsley.
3. In a small bowl, whisk together olive oil, lemon juice, Dijon mustard, minced garlic, salt, and pepper to create the dressing.
4. Pour the dressing over the quinoa mixture and toss until well combined.
5. Adjust seasoning to taste.
6. Chill in the refrigerator for at least 15 minutes before serving to allow flavors to meld.
7. Serve the quinoa salad chilled and enjoy a nutritious and flavorful meal!

Turkey and Avocado Wrap

Serving: 1 wrap **Preparation Time**: 10 minutes **Total Time:** 10 minutes

Ingredients:

- 1 wholegrain or spinach tortilla
- 46 slices of turkey breast
- $\frac{1}{2}$ avocado, sliced
- $\frac{1}{4}$ cup cherry tomatoes, halved
- $\frac{1}{4}$ cup cucumber, thinly sliced
- 1 tablespoon Greek yogurt or mayonnaise

- Fresh lettuce leaves
- Salt and pepper to taste

Instructions:

1. Lay the tortilla flat on a clean surface.
2. Arrange the turkey slices evenly across the tortilla.
3. Layer avocado slices, cherry tomatoes, and cucumber on top of the turkey.
4. Spread Greek yogurt or mayonnaise over the veggies.
5. Place fresh lettuce leaves on the spread.
6. Season with salt and pepper to taste.
7. Carefully fold the sides of the tortilla inward and roll it up tightly to form a wrap.
8. Slice the wrap in half diagonally if desired.
9. Serve immediately and enjoy a quick and satisfying Turkey and Avocado Wrap!

Lentil Soup

Serving: 4 servings **Preparation Time:** 15 minutes **Cooking Time:** 1hr **Total Time:** 1hr 15 minutes

Ingredients:

- 1 cup dried lentils, rinsed and drained
- 1 onion, finely chopped
- 2 carrots, diced
- 2 celery stalks, chopped
- 3 cloves garlic, minced
- 1 can (14 oz) diced tomatoes

- 6 cups vegetable broth
- 1 teaspoon ground cumin
- 1 teaspoon ground coriander
- $^1/_2$ teaspoon smoked paprika
- 1 bay leaf
- Salt and pepper to taste
- 2 tablespoons olive oil
- Fresh lemon wedges (for serving)

Instructions:

1. In a large pot, heat olive oil over medium heat. Add chopped onion, carrots, and celery. Sauté until vegetables are softened, about 5 minutes.
2. Add minced garlic, ground cumin, ground coriander, smoked paprika, and continue sautéing for an additional 2 minutes.
3. Pour in diced tomatoes (with juices) and vegetable broth. Add rinsed lentils and the bay leaf. Bring to a boil.
4. Reduce heat to low, cover, and simmer for 45 min minutes or until lentils are tender.
5. Season with salt and pepper to taste.
6. Remove the bay leaf before serving.
7. Squeeze fresh lemon juice into each bowl before serving for a burst of flavor.

Chickpea and Spinach Curry

Serving: 4 servings **Preparation Time:** 15 minutes **Cooking Time:** 25 minutes **Total Time:** 40 minutes

---

Ingredients:

- 2 cans (15 oz each) chickpeas, drained and rinsed
- 1 onion, finely chopped
- 3 cloves garlic, minced
- 1 inch ginger, grated
- 1 can (14 oz) diced tomatoes
- 1 can (14 oz) coconut milk
- 4 cups fresh spinach leaves
- 2 tablespoons curry powder
- 1 teaspoon ground cumin
- 1 teaspoon ground coriander
- $^1/_2$ teaspoon turmeric
- $^1/_2$ teaspoon cayenne pepper (optional, for heat)
- Salt and pepper to taste
- 2 tablespoons vegetable oil
- Fresh cilantro, chopped (for garnish)
- Cooked rice or naan (for serving)

Instructions:

1. In a large pan, heat vegetable oil over medium heat. Add chopped onion and cook until softened.
2. Add minced garlic and grated ginger, sauté for an additional 12 minutes.
3. Stir in curry powder, ground cumin, ground coriander, turmeric, and cayenne pepper (if using). Cook for 12 minutes to toast the spices.
4. Pour in diced tomatoes (with juices) and coconut milk. Bring to a simmer.
5. Add drained chickpeas and continue simmering for 1520 minutes, allowing the flavors to meld.
6. Stir in fresh spinach until wilted.
7. Season with salt and pepper to taste.
8. Serve the Chickpea and Spinach Curry over cooked rice or with naan.
9. Garnish with fresh cilantro before serving.

Grilled Salmon Salad

Serving: 2 **Preparation Time:** 10 minutes **Cooking Time:** 10 minutes
Total Time: 20 minutes

Ingredients:

- 2 salmon filets
- Salt and pepper to taste
- 6 cups mixed salad greens
- 1 cup cherry tomatoes, halved
- 1 cucumber, sliced
- 1/4 red onion, thinly sliced
- 2 tablespoons extra-virgin olive oil
- 1 tablespoon balsamic vinegar
- 1 teaspoon Dijon mustard
- Fresh lemon wedges for serving

Instructions:

1. Preheat the grill to medium-high heat.
2. Season the salmon filets with salt and pepper.
3. Grill the salmon for about 4-5 minutes per side, or until it flakes easily with a fork.
4. In a large bowl, toss together the mixed salad greens, cherry tomatoes, cucumber, and red onion.
5. In a small bowl, whisk together the olive oil, balsamic vinegar, and Dijon mustard to create the dressing.
6. Place the grilled salmon filets on top of the salad.
7. Drizzle the salad with the prepared dressing.
8. Serve immediately, garnishing with fresh lemon wedges.

Mediterranean Chickpea Salad

Serving: 4 **Preparation Time:** 15 minutes

Ingredients:

- 2 cans (15 oz each) chickpeas, drained and rinsed
- 1 cup cherry tomatoes, halved
- 1 cucumber, diced
- $1/2$ red onion, finely chopped
- $1/2$ cup feta cheese, crumbled
- $1/4$ cup Kalamata olives, pitted and sliced
- $1/4$ cup fresh parsley, chopped
- 2 tablespoons extra-virgin olive oil
- 2 tablespoons red wine vinegar
- 1 teaspoon dried oregano
- Salt and pepper to taste

Instructions:

1. In a large bowl, combine the chickpeas, cherry tomatoes, cucumber, red onion, feta cheese, olives, and parsley.
2. In a small bowl, whisk together the olive oil, red wine vinegar, dried oregano, salt, and pepper to create the dressing.
3. Pour the dressing over the chickpea mixture and toss gently until all ingredients are well coated.
4. Adjust salt and pepper to taste.
5. Serve immediately or refrigerate for a couple of hours before serving to allow flavors to meld.

Greek Yogurt Chicken Salad

Serving: 2 Preparation Time: 15 minutes

Ingredients:

- 2 boneless, skinless chicken breasts, cooked and diced
- $1/2$ cup Greek yogurt
- $1/4$ cup cucumber, diced
- $1/4$ cup cherry tomatoes, halved
- $1/4$ cup red onion, finely chopped
- 2 tablespoons feta cheese, crumbled
- 1 tablespoon Kalamata olives, pitted and sliced
- 1 tablespoon fresh dill, chopped
- 1 tablespoon extra-virgin olive oil
- 1 teaspoon lemon juice
- Salt and pepper to taste
- Whole grain pita bread or salad greens for serving

Instructions:

1. In a large bowl, combine the diced chicken, Greek yogurt, cucumber, cherry tomatoes, red onion, feta cheese, olives, and fresh dill.
2. In a small bowl, whisk together the olive oil and lemon juice.
3. Pour the dressing over the chicken mixture and toss gently until well coated.
4. Season with salt and pepper to taste.
5. Serve the Greek Yogurt Chicken Salad on whole grain pita bread or a bed of salad greens.

Roasted Vegetable Quinoa Bowl

Serving: 2 **Preparation Time:** 15 minutes **Cooking Time:** 25 minutes
Total Time: 40 minutes

Ingredients:

- 1 cup quinoa, rinsed
- 2 cups mixed vegetables (e.g., bell peppers, zucchini, cherry tomatoes)
- 1 red onion, sliced
- 2 tablespoons olive oil
- 1 teaspoon dried oregano
- 1 teaspoon smoked paprika
- Salt and pepper to taste
- $^{1}/_{4}$ cup feta cheese, crumbled
- Fresh parsley for garnish
- **Optional:** Balsamic glaze for drizzling

Instructions:

1. Preheat the oven to 425°F (220°C).
2. In a bowl, toss the mixed vegetables and red onion with olive oil, dried oregano, smoked paprika, salt, and pepper.
3. Spread the vegetables on a baking sheet in a single layer.
4. Roast in the preheated oven for about 20-25 minutes, or until the vegetables are tender and slightly caramelized, stirring halfway through.
5. While the vegetables are roasting, cook the quinoa according to package instructions.
6. Once the quinoa and vegetables are ready, assemble the bowls by placing a serving of quinoa in each bowl.

7. Top with the roasted vegetables, crumbled feta cheese, and fresh parsley.
8. **Optional:** Drizzle with balsamic glaze for added flavor.
9. Serve warm and enjoy your Roasted Vegetable Quinoa Bowl!

This bowl is not only visually appealing but also a nutritious and satisfying meal.

Whole Wheat Pasta Primavera

Serving: 4 **Preparation Time:** 15 minutes **Cooking Time:** 15 minutes
Total Time: 30 minutes

Ingredients:

- 8 ounces whole wheat pasta
- 2 tablespoons olive oil
- 2 cloves garlic, minced
- 1 cup cherry tomatoes, halved
- 1 medium zucchini, thinly sliced
- 1 medium carrot, julienned
- 1 bell pepper, thinly sliced
- 1 cup broccoli florets
- Salt and pepper to taste
- $1/2$ teaspoon dried oregano
- $1/2$ teaspoon dried basil
- $1/4$ cup grated Parmesan cheese
- Fresh basil or parsley for garnish

Instructions:

1. Cook the whole wheat pasta according to package instructions. Drain and set aside.
2. In a large skillet, heat olive oil over medium heat. Add minced garlic and sauté until fragrant.
3. Add cherry tomatoes, zucchini, carrot, bell pepper, and broccoli to the skillet. Sauté for about 5-7 minutes until the vegetables are tender-crisp.
4. Season the vegetables with salt, pepper, dried oregano, and dried basil. Stir to combine.
5. Add the cooked pasta to the skillet and toss everything together until well mixed.
6. Cook for an additional 2-3 minutes, allowing the flavors to meld.
7. Sprinkle grated Parmesan cheese over the pasta and vegetables. Toss again.
8. Garnish with fresh basil or parsley.
9. Serve warm and enjoy your Whole Wheat Pasta Primavera!

Salmon and Asparagus Foil Packets

Serving: 2 **Preparation Time:** 10 minutes **Cooking Time:** 20 minutes
Total Time: 30 minutes

Ingredients:

- 2 salmon filets
- 1 bunch asparagus, tough ends trimmed
- 2 tablespoons olive oil
- 2 cloves garlic, minced

- 1 lemon, sliced
- Salt and pepper to taste
- Fresh dill for garnish

Instructions:

1. Preheat the oven to 400°F (200°C).
2. Place each salmon filet in the center of a large piece of aluminum foil.
3. Arrange asparagus spears around each salmon filet.
4. Drizzle olive oil over the salmon and asparagus. Sprinkle minced garlic evenly over each filet.
5. Season with salt and pepper to taste.
6. Place lemon slices on top of each salmon filet.
7. Fold the sides of the foil over the salmon and asparagus, creating a sealed packet.
8. Place the foil packets on a baking sheet and bake in the preheated oven for about 18-20 minutes, or until the salmon is cooked through and flakes easily with a fork.
9. Carefully open the foil packets, garnish with fresh dill, and serve.

This Salmon and Asparagus Foil Packets recipe is not only delicious but also a convenient and healthy way to prepare a complete meal in one go. Enjoy!

Quinoa Stuffed Bell Peppers

Serving: 4 **Preparation Time:** 15 minutes **Cooking Time:** 25 minutes **Total Time:** 40 minutes

Ingredients:

- 4 large bell peppers, halved and seeds removed
- 1 cup quinoa, rinsed
- 2 cups vegetable broth or water
- 1 tablespoon olive oil
- 1 onion, finely chopped
- 2 cloves garlic, minced
- 1 zucchini, diced
- 1 carrot, grated
- 1 can (15 oz) black beans, drained and rinsed
- 1 cup corn kernels (fresh or frozen)
- 1 teaspoon ground cumin
- 1 teaspoon chili powder
- Salt and pepper to taste
- 1 cup shredded cheese (cheddar or your choice)
- Fresh cilantro or parsley for garnish

Instructions:

1. Preheat the oven to 375°F (190°C).
2. In a saucepan, combine quinoa and vegetable broth (or water). Bring to a boil, then reduce heat, cover, and simmer for 15-20 minutes, or until quinoa is cooked and liquid is absorbed.
3. While quinoa is cooking, heat olive oil in a large skillet over medium heat. Add chopped onion and garlic, sauté until softened.
4. Add diced zucchini, grated carrot, black beans, corn, ground cumin, chili powder, salt, and pepper to the skillet. Cook for 5-7 minutes until vegetables are tender.
5. Combine the cooked quinoa with the vegetable mixture, stirring well to combine.
6. Place bell pepper halves in a baking dish. Fill each pepper half with the quinoa and vegetable mixture.
7. Top each stuffed pepper with shredded cheese.
8. Bake in the preheated oven for about 20-25 minutes, or until the peppers are tender and the cheese is melted and bubbly.
9. Garnish with fresh cilantro or parsley before serving.

Caprese Salad with Whole Wheat Pita

Serving: 2 Preparation Time: 10 minutes

Ingredients:

- 2 whole wheat pita bread, cut into wedges
- 2 large tomatoes, sliced
- 1 ball fresh mozzarella cheese, sliced
- Fresh basil leaves
- 2 tablespoons extra-virgin olive oil
- Balsamic glaze for drizzling
- Salt and pepper to taste

Instructions:

1. Preheat the oven to 375°F (190°C).
2. Place whole wheat pita wedges on a baking sheet. Bake in the preheated oven for about 8-10 minutes, or until they are crispy and golden brown.
3. While the pita is baking, arrange sliced tomatoes and fresh mozzarella alternately on a serving plate.
4. Tuck fresh basil leaves between the tomato and mozzarella slices.
5. Drizzle extra-virgin olive oil over the tomato and mozzarella slices.
6. Season with salt and pepper to taste.
7. Once the whole wheat pita wedges are ready, arrange them around the edges of the plate.
8. Drizzle balsamic glaze over the Caprese salad just before serving.
9. Serve immediately and enjoy your Caprese Salad with Whole Wheat Pita!

Tuna and White Bean Salad

Serving: 2 **Preparation Time:** 10 minutes

Ingredients:

- 1 can (15 oz) white beans, drained and rinsed
- 1 can (5 oz) tuna, drained
- $\frac{1}{2}$ red onion, finely chopped
- 1 celery stalk, diced
- $\frac{1}{4}$ cup fresh parsley, chopped
- 2 tablespoons capers, drained
- 2 tablespoons extra-virgin olive oil
- 1 tablespoon red wine vinegar
- Salt and pepper to taste
- **Optional:** Lemon wedges for serving

Instructions:

1. In a large bowl, combine the white beans, tuna, red onion, celery, parsley, and capers.
2. In a small bowl, whisk together the olive oil and red wine vinegar.
3. Pour the dressing over the tuna and white bean mixture.
4. Toss gently to combine all ingredients and coat them evenly with the dressing.
5. Season with salt and pepper to taste.
6. **Optional:** Serve with lemon wedges on the side for extra freshness.
7. Refrigerate for a short time before serving if you prefer a chilled salad.

Eggplant and Tomato Ratatouille

Serving: 4 **Preparation Time:** 15 minutes **Cooking Time:** 25 minutes
Total Time: 40 minutes

Ingredients:

- 1 large eggplant, diced
- 2 zucchini, sliced
- 1 bell pepper, diced
- 1 onion, finely chopped
- 3 cloves garlic, minced
- 1 can (14 oz) diced tomatoes, undrained
- 1 can (6 oz) tomato paste
- 2 tablespoons olive oil
- 1 teaspoon dried thyme
- 1 teaspoon dried rosemary
- Salt and pepper to taste
- Fresh basil or parsley for garnish

Instructions:

1. In a large skillet or pot, heat olive oil over medium heat.
2. Add chopped onion and minced garlic. Sauté until the onion is translucent.
3. Add diced eggplant, zucchini, and bell pepper to the skillet. Cook for about 5-7 minutes until the vegetables start to soften.
4. Stir in diced tomatoes and tomato paste. Mix well.
5. Season with dried thyme, dried rosemary, salt, and pepper. Stir to combine.
6. Reduce the heat to low, cover, and let the ratatouille simmer for about 15-20 minutes, or until the vegetables are tender.
7. Garnish with fresh basil or parsley before serving.

6

DINNER DELIGHT

Baked Salmon with Lemon and Herbs

Serving: 4 servings **Preparation Time**: 10 minutes **Baking Time:** 1520 minutes **Total Time:** 2530 minutes

---

Ingredients:

- 4 salmon filets
- 2 tablespoons olive oil
- 2 tablespoons fresh lemon juice
- Zest of one lemon
- cloves garlic, minced
- 1 teaspoon dried oregano
- 1 teaspoon dried thyme
- Salt and pepper to taste
- Lemon slices (for garnish)
- Fresh herbs (such as parsley or dill, for garnish)

Instructions:

1. Preheat the oven to 375°F (190°C).
2. Place the salmon filets on a baking sheet lined with parchment paper.
3. In a bowl, mix together olive oil, fresh lemon juice, lemon zest, minced garlic, dried oregano, dried thyme, salt, and pepper.
4. Brush the lemon and herb mixture over the salmon filets, ensuring they are evenly coated.
5. Bake in the preheated oven for 1520 minutes or until the salmon is cooked through and flakes easily with a fork.

6. Garnish with lemon slices and fresh herbs.
7. Serve the Baked Salmon with Lemon and Herbs with your favorite side dishes.

Grilled Chicken Breast with Roasted Vegetables

Serving: 4 **Preparation Time:** 15 minutes **Marinating Time:** 30 minutes (optional) **Grilling Time:** 15-20 minutes **Roasting Time:** 25-30 minutes **Total Time:** 1 hour 30 minutes (including marinating time and resting)

Ingredients:

- 4 boneless, skinless chicken breasts
- 2 tablespoons olive oil
- 2 tablespoons balsamic vinegar
- 2 tablespoons honey or maple syrup
- 2 cloves garlic, minced
- 1 teaspoon dried thyme
- Salt and pepper to taste

For Roasted Vegetables:

- 1 lb (450g) mixed vegetables (e.g., bell peppers, zucchini, cherry tomatoes, carrots), chopped
- 2 tablespoons olive oil
- Salt and pepper to taste
- Fresh herbs (such as parsley or thyme, for garnish)

Instructions:

1. In a bowl, whisk together olive oil, balsamic vinegar, honey or maple syrup, minced garlic, dried thyme, salt, and pepper to create the marinade.
2. Place chicken breasts in a dish and pour half of the marinade over them. Let them marinate for at least 30 minutes in the refrigerator (optional).
3. Preheat the grill to medium-high heat.
4. Remove chicken from the refrigerator and let it come to room temperature for about 10 minutes.
5. Grill the chicken breasts for 6-8 minutes per side or until fully cooked and juices run clear. Ensure an internal temperature of 165°F (74°C).
6. While the chicken is grilling, preheat the oven to 400°F (200°C).
7. Toss chopped vegetables with olive oil, salt, and pepper. Spread them on a baking sheet.
8. Roast the vegetables in the preheated oven for 25-30 minutes or until they are tender and slightly caramelized.
9. Rest the grilled chicken for a few minutes before slicing.
10. Serve the Grilled Chicken Breast with Roasted Vegetables, garnished with fresh herbs.

Spaghetti Squash Primavera

Serving: 4 **Preparation Time:** 15 minutes **Cooking Time:** 45 minutes
Total Time: 1 hour

Ingredients:

- 1 medium-sized spaghetti squash
- 2 tablespoons olive oil

- 1 teaspoon dried oregano
- 1 teaspoon dried basil
- Salt and pepper to taste

For Primavera Sauce:

- 2 tablespoons olive oil
- 1 onion, thinly sliced
- 2 cloves garlic, minced
- 1 bell pepper, thinly sliced
- 1 zucchini, thinly sliced
- 1 carrot, julienned
- 1 cup cherry tomatoes, halved
- $\frac{1}{2}$ cup frozen peas
- $\frac{1}{4}$ cup fresh basil, chopped
- Salt and pepper to taste
- Grated Parmesan cheese (optional, for serving)

Instructions:

1. Preheat the oven to 400°F (200°C).
2. Cut the spaghetti squash in half lengthwise. Scoop out the seeds and fibers.
3. Brush the inside of each squash half with olive oil, then sprinkle with dried oregano, dried basil, salt, and pepper.
4. Place the squash halves on a baking sheet, cut side down. Roast in the preheated oven for 35-40 minutes or until the squash is tender and easily pierced with a fork.
5. While the squash is roasting, prepare the primavera sauce. In a large pan, heat olive oil over medium heat. Add sliced onion, minced garlic, bell pepper, zucchini, and julienned carrot. Sauté until the vegetables are tender-crisp.
6. Stir in cherry tomatoes and frozen peas. Cook for an additional 2-3 minutes.

7. Once the spaghetti squash is cooked, use a fork to scrape the flesh into spaghetti-like strands.
8. Add the spaghetti squash strands to the pan with the sautéed vegetables. Toss everything together until well combined.
9. Season with salt and pepper to taste. Stir in fresh basil.
10. Serve the Spaghetti Squash Primavera hot, optionally topped with grated Parmesan cheese.

Teriyaki Tofu Stir-Fry

Serving: 4   **Preparation Time:** 15 minutes **Marinating Time:** 30 minutes (optional)   **Cooking Time:** 15 minutes **Total Time:** 1 hour (including marinating time)

Ingredients:

- 14 oz (400g) firm tofu, pressed and cubed
- $1/4$ cup soy sauce
- 2 tablespoons rice vinegar
- 2 tablespoons mirin (sweet rice wine)
- 2 tablespoons honey or maple syrup
- 1 tablespoon sesame oil
- 2 cloves garlic, minced
- 1 teaspoon fresh ginger, grated
- 2 tablespoons vegetable oil
- 1 red bell pepper, sliced
- 1 yellow bell pepper, sliced
- 1 broccoli crown, cut into florets
- 1 carrot, julienned
- 2 cups snap peas, ends trimmed
- 2 green onions, sliced (for garnish)

- Sesame seeds (for garnish)
- Cooked rice or noodles (for serving)

Instructions:

1. Press tofu to remove excess moisture, then cut it into cubes.
2. In a bowl, whisk together soy sauce, rice vinegar, mirin, honey or maple syrup, sesame oil, minced garlic, and grated ginger to make the teriyaki sauce.
3. Place tofu cubes in a dish and pour half of the teriyaki sauce over them. Let it marinate for at least 30 minutes in the refrigerator (optional).
4. Heat vegetable oil in a wok or large pan over medium-high heat.
5. Add marinated tofu and cook until golden brown on all sides. Remove from the pan and set aside.
6. In the same pan, add a bit more oil if needed. Stir-fry bell peppers, broccoli, carrot, and snap peas until they are crisp-tender.
7. Return the cooked tofu to the pan and pour the remaining teriyaki sauce over the tofu and vegetables. Stir to coat evenly and heat through.
8. Serve the Teriyaki Tofu Stir-Fry over cooked rice or noodles.
9. Garnish with sliced green onions and sesame seeds.

This flavorful and vegetarian Teriyaki Tofu Stir-Fry is a delicious and wholesome meal. Enjoy!

Baked Cod with Tomato Basil Salsa

Serving: 4 **Preparation Time:** 15 minutes **Baking Time:** 15-20 minutes **Total Time:** 35 minutes

---

Ingredients:

- 4 cod filets
- 2 tablespoons olive oil
- 1 teaspoon dried oregano
- 1 teaspoon smoked paprika
- Salt and pepper to taste

For **Tomato Basil Salsa:**

- 1 cup cherry tomatoes, quartered
- $^1/_4$ cup fresh basil, chopped
- 2 tablespoons red onion, finely chopped
- 1 tablespoon balsamic vinegar
- 1 tablespoon olive oil
- Salt and pepper to taste

Instructions:

1. Preheat the oven to 400°F (200°C).
2. Pat the cod filets dry with paper towels and place them on a baking sheet.
3. In a small bowl, mix together olive oil, dried oregano, smoked paprika, salt, and pepper. Brush the mixture over the cod filets.
4. Bake in the preheated oven for 15-20 minutes or until the cod is opaque and flakes easily with a fork.
5. While the cod is baking, prepare the tomato basil salsa by combining quartered cherry tomatoes, chopped fresh basil, finely chopped red onion, balsamic vinegar, olive oil, salt, and pepper in a bowl. Toss gently to combine.
6. Once the cod is done, remove it from the oven and transfer it to serving plates.
7. Spoon the Tomato Basil Salsa over the baked cod filets.
8. Serve the Baked Cod with Tomato Basil Salsa with your favorite side dishes.

Balsamic Glazed Brussels Sprouts with Quinoa

Serving: 4 **Preparation Time:** 15 minutes **Cooking Time:** 25 minutes
Total Time: 40 minutes

Ingredients:

- 1 cup quinoa, rinsed
- 2 cups Brussels sprouts, trimmed and halved
- 2 tablespoons olive oil
- 2 tablespoons balsamic vinegar
- 1 tablespoon honey or maple syrup
- 2 cloves garlic, minced
- Salt and pepper to taste
- Optional: Crushed red pepper flakes for a hint of spice
- $1/4$ cup chopped walnuts (optional, for garnish)
- Fresh parsley for garnish

Instructions:

1. Cook quinoa according to package instructions. Set aside.
2. Preheat the oven to 400°F (200°C).
3. In a bowl, toss Brussels sprouts with olive oil, balsamic vinegar, honey (or maple syrup), minced garlic, salt, and pepper.
4. Spread the Brussels sprouts evenly on a baking sheet lined with parchment paper.
5. Roast in the preheated oven for about 20-25 minutes, or until the Brussels sprouts are caramelized and tender, stirring halfway through.
6. While the Brussels sprouts are roasting, fluff the cooked quinoa with a fork.
7. Once the Brussels sprouts are done, mix them with the cooked quinoa in a serving bowl.
8. If desired, sprinkle with crushed red pepper flakes for a touch of heat.

9. Garnish with chopped walnuts (if using) and fresh parsley.
10. Serve warm and enjoy your Balsamic Glazed Brussels Sprouts with Quinoa!

This dish offers a perfect balance of sweetness from the balsamic glaze, nuttiness from the quinoa, and a delightful crunch if you choose to add walnuts. It's a nutritious and flavorful option for a DASH diet dinner.

Farro and Roasted Vegetable Bowl

Serving: 4 **Preparation Time:** 15 minutes **Cooking Time:** 25 minutes **Total Time:** 40 minutes

Ingredients:

- 1 cup farro, rinsed
- 2 cups mixed vegetables (e.g., Brussels sprouts, carrots, bell peppers), chopped
- 2 tablespoons olive oil
- 1 teaspoon dried thyme
- 1 teaspoon dried rosemary
- Salt and pepper to taste
- 1 cup cherry tomatoes, halved
- $\frac{1}{4}$ cup crumbled feta cheese (optional)
- Balsamic glaze for drizzling
- Fresh basil or parsley for garnish

Instructions:

1. Cook farro according to package instructions. Set aside.
2. Preheat the oven to 400°F (200°C).

3. In a bowl, toss mixed vegetables with olive oil, dried thyme, dried rosemary, salt, and pepper.
4. Spread the vegetables on a baking sheet lined with parchment paper.
5. Roast in the preheated oven for about 20-25 minutes, or until the vegetables are tender and slightly caramelized, stirring halfway through.
6. While the vegetables are roasting, fluff the cooked farro with a fork.
7. Once the vegetables are done, assemble the bowls by placing a serving of farro in each bowl.
8. Top with the roasted vegetables, cherry tomatoes, and crumbled feta cheese (if using).
9. Drizzle with balsamic glaze and garnish with fresh basil or parsley.
10. Serve warm and enjoy your Farro and Roasted Vegetable Bowl!

Honey Mustard Glazed Turkey Meatballs

Serving: 4 servings **Preparation Time:** 15 minutes **Cooking Time:** 20 minutes **Total Time:** 35 minutes

Ingredients:

- For the Turkey Meatballs:
- 1 pound ground turkey
- $1/2$ cup breadcrumbs
- $1/4$ cup grated Parmesan cheese
- 1 egg
- 2 cloves garlic, minced
- 1 teaspoon dried oregano
- Salt and pepper to taste
- Olive oil for cooking

For the **Honey Mustard Glaze:**

- $^1/_4$ cup Dijon mustard
- 2 tablespoons honey
- 1 tablespoon apple cider vinegar
- 1 teaspoon soy sauce

Instructions:

1. Preheat the oven to 375°F (190°C).
2. In a bowl, combine ground turkey, breadcrumbs, Parmesan cheese, egg, minced garlic, dried oregano, salt, and pepper. Mix until well combined.
3. Form the mixture into small meatballs and place them on a baking sheet lined with parchment paper.
4. Heat olive oil in a skillet over medium-high heat. Brown the meatballs on all sides until cooked through, but not completely done.
5. Transfer the partially cooked meatballs to the preheated oven and bake for an additional 10-12 minutes, or until they are fully cooked and have a golden-brown color.
6. While the meatballs are baking, prepare the honey mustard glaze by whisking together Dijon mustard, honey, apple cider vinegar, and soy sauce in a small bowl.
7. Once the meatballs are done, remove them from the oven and brush them with the honey mustard glaze.
8. Serve the glazed turkey meatballs warm, and optionally, garnish with chopped fresh parsley.

Pomegranate Glazed Chicken

Serving: 4 servings **Preparation Time:** 15 minutes **Cooking Time:** 25 minutes **Total Time:** 40 minutes

---

Ingredients:

- 4 boneless, skinless chicken breasts
- Salt and pepper to taste
- 1 tablespoon olive oil
- 1/2 cup pomegranate juice
- 1/4 cup balsamic vinegar
- 2 tablespoons honey
- 1 teaspoon Dijon mustard
- 2 cloves garlic, minced
- 1 teaspoon fresh thyme leaves (or 1/2 teaspoon dried thyme)
- Fresh pomegranate arils for garnish (optional)
- Fresh parsley for garnish

Instructions:

1. Preheat the oven to 375°F (190°C).
2. Season chicken breasts with salt and pepper on both sides.
3. In an oven-safe skillet, heat olive oil over medium-high heat.
4. Sear the chicken breasts for 3-4 minutes per side until they develop a golden-brown crust.
5. In a bowl, whisk together pomegranate juice, balsamic vinegar, honey, Dijon mustard, minced garlic, and thyme.
6. Pour the pomegranate glaze over the seared chicken breasts in the skillet.
7. Transfer the skillet to the preheated oven and bake for 20-25 minutes or until the chicken is cooked through.

8. Baste the chicken with the glaze every 10 minutes to ensure a flavorful coating.
9. Garnish with fresh pomegranate arils and parsley before serving.
10.   Serve the Pomegranate Glazed Chicken over a bed of quinoa, rice, or your preferred whole grain.

Harvest Chicken Skillet

Serving: 4 **Preparation Time:** 15 minutes **Cooking Time:** 25 minutes **Total Time:** 40 minutes

---

Ingredients:

- 4 boneless, skinless chicken breasts
- Salt and pepper to taste
- 2 tablespoons olive oil
- 1 cup Brussels sprouts, trimmed and halved
- 1 cup butternut squash, peeled and diced
- $\frac{1}{2}$ cup dried cranberries
- $\frac{1}{4}$ cup chopped pecans
- 2 tablespoons maple syrup
- 1 tablespoon Dijon mustard
- 1 teaspoon dried thyme
- $\frac{1}{2}$ teaspoon ground cinnamon
- Fresh parsley for garnish

Instructions:

1. Preheat the oven to 375°F (190°C).
2. Season chicken breasts with salt and pepper on both sides.
3. In an oven-safe skillet, heat olive oil over medium-high heat.

4. Sear the chicken breasts for 3-4 minutes per side until they develop a golden-brown crust. Remove from the skillet and set aside.
5. In the same skillet, add Brussels sprouts and butternut squash. Sauté for 3-4 minutes until slightly softened.
6. In a small bowl, whisk together maple syrup, Dijon mustard, dried thyme, and ground cinnamon.
7. Add dried cranberries and chopped pecans to the skillet with the vegetables.
8. Return the seared chicken breasts to the skillet and pour the maple-Dijon mixture over everything.
9. Transfer the skillet to the preheated oven and bake for 20-25 minutes or until the chicken is cooked through.
10. Garnish with fresh parsley before serving.

7

SNACKS & APPETIZERS

Hummus with Veggies

Serving: 4 servings **Preparation Time:** 10 minutes **Time:** 10 minutes

---

Ingredients:

- 1 cup hummus (store-bought or homemade)
- Assorted vegetables for dipping (carrot sticks, cucumber slices, bell pepper strips, cherry tomatoes, etc.)
- Olive oil (optional, for drizzling)
- Paprika or cumin (optional, for garnish)
- Fresh parsley or cilantro (optional, for garnish)

Instructions:

1. Arrange the assorted vegetables on a serving platter or individual plates.
2. Place a bowl of hummus in the center of the platter or on each plate.
3. Optionally, drizzle a bit of olive oil over the hummus for added richness.
4. Sprinkle a pinch of paprika or cumin on top of the hummus for extra flavor (optional).
5. Garnish with fresh parsley or cilantro for a pop of color (optional).
6. Serve immediately and enjoy this healthy and flavorful Hummus with Veggies as a snack or appetizer.

Greek Yogurt Dip

Serving: 4 **Preparation Time:** 10 minutes **Total Time:** 10 minutes

---

Ingredients:

- 1 cup Greek yogurt
- 1 cucumber, finely diced
- 1 clove garlic, minced
- 1 tablespoon fresh dill, chopped
- 1 tablespoon fresh mint, chopped
- 1 tablespoon lemon juice
- Salt and pepper to taste
- Olive oil (optional, for drizzling)
- Whole grain pita bread or vegetable sticks (for serving)

Instructions:

1. In a bowl, combine Greek yogurt, diced cucumber, minced garlic, chopped dill, chopped mint, and lemon juice.
2. Season the mixture with salt and pepper to taste. Stir well to combine.
3. Optionally, drizzle a bit of olive oil over the top for extra richness.
4. Refrigerate the Greek Yogurt Dip for at least 30 minutes to allow the flavors to meld.
5. 5. Before serving, give the dip a final stir and adjust the seasoning if needed.
6. Serve the Greek Yogurt Dip with whole grain pita bread or vegetable sticks.
7. Enjoy this refreshing and creamy dip as a healthy snack or appetizer.

Fresh Fruit Salsa with Whole Grain Chips

Serving: 4 **Preparation Time:** 15 minutes **Total Time:** 15 minutes

Ingredients:

- 1 cup diced fresh pineapple
- 1 cup diced strawberries
- 1 mango, peeled and diced
- 1 kiwi, peeled and diced
- $^1/_2$ cup blueberries
- 1 tablespoon honey or maple syrup
- 1 tablespoon fresh lime juice
- 1 tablespoon fresh mint, chopped
- Whole grain tortilla chips or pita chips

Instructions:

1. In a large bowl, combine diced pineapple, strawberries, mango, kiwi, and blueberries.
2. Drizzle honey or maple syrup over the fruit.
3. Add fresh lime juice and chopped mint. Gently toss to combine.
4. Allow the fruit salsa to sit for a few minutes to let the flavors meld.
5. Serve the Fresh Fruit Salsa in a bowl alongside whole grain tortilla chips or pita chips.
6. Enjoy this vibrant and refreshing snack!

Mango Salsa with Cinnamon Tortilla Chips

Serving: 4 **Preparation Time:** 15 minutes **Total Time:** 15 minutes

Ingredients:

- For Mango Salsa:
- 2 ripe mangoes, peeled and diced
- $^1/_2$ red onion, finely chopped
- 1 red bell pepper, diced
- 1 jalapeño, seeds removed and finely chopped
- $^1/_4$ cup fresh cilantro, chopped
- Juice of 2 limes
- Salt to taste

For **Cinnamon Tortilla Chips:**

- 4 whole wheat or corn tortillas
- 1 tablespoon olive oil
- 1 tablespoon sugar
- 1 teaspoon ground cinnamon

Instructions:

For **Mango Salsa:**

1. In a bowl, combine diced mangoes, chopped red onion, diced red bell pepper, chopped jalapeño, chopped cilantro, and lime juice.
2. Season with salt to taste. Gently toss to combine.
3. Allow the Mango Salsa to sit for a few minutes to enhance flavors.

For **Cinnamon Tortilla Chips:**

1. Preheat the oven to 350°F (180°C).
2. Brush each tortilla with olive oil on both sides.
3. In a small bowl, mix together sugar and ground cinnamon.
4. Sprinkle the cinnamon-sugar mixture over the tortillas.
5. Stack the tortillas and cut them into wedges.

6. Arrange the tortilla wedges on a baking sheet in a single layer.
7. Bake in the preheated oven for 8-10 minutes or until the chips are crisp and golden.
8. Allow the cinnamon tortilla chips to cool before serving.

Serve the *Mango Salsa* with *Cinnamon Tortilla Chips*:

1. Serve the Mango Salsa in a bowl alongside the cinnamon tortilla chips.
2. Enjoy this delightful and fruity salsa with the sweet crunch of cinnamon tortilla chips.

Cottage Cheese with Pineapple Recipe:

Servings: 2 **Preparation Time:** 5 minutes **Total Time:** 5 minutes

Ingredients:

- 1 cup cottage cheese
- 1 cup fresh pineapple chunks
- 2 tablespoons honey (optional)
- $^{1}/_{4}$ cup chopped nuts (e.g., almonds or walnuts, optional)

Instructions:

1. In a bowl, combine cottage cheese and fresh pineapple chunks.
2. If you prefer a touch of sweetness, drizzle honey over the mixture.
3. Optionally, sprinkle chopped nuts on top for added crunch and flavor.

4. Gently toss the ingredients together until well combined.
5. Divide the Cottage Cheese with Pineapple into serving bowls.
6. Serve immediately and enjoy this quick and satisfying snack or breakfast option.

Tuna Lettuce Wraps Recipe:

Servings: 2 **Preparation Time:** 10 minutes **Total Time:** 15 minutes

---

Ingredients:

- 1 can (5 oz) tuna, drained
- $\frac{1}{4}$ cup red onion, finely chopped
- $\frac{1}{4}$ cup celery, finely chopped
- 2 tablespoons mayonnaise
- 1 tablespoon Dijon mustard
- Salt and pepper to taste
- 4 large lettuce leaves (e.g., iceberg or butter lettuce)
- Tomato slices and avocado (optional, for garnish)

Instructions:

1. In a bowl, combine drained tuna, chopped red onion, chopped celery, mayonnaise, and Dijon mustard.
2. Mix the ingredients until well combined.
3. Season with salt and pepper to taste.
4. Spoon the tuna mixture onto the center of each lettuce leaf.
5. **Optional:** Garnish with tomato slices and avocado.
6. Fold the sides of the lettuce leaf over the tuna mixture to create a wrap.
7. Secure with toothpicks if needed.

8. Serve the Tuna Lettuce Wraps immediately and enjoy this light and protein-packed meal.

Baked Zucchini Chips Recipe:

Servings: 4 **Preparation Time:** 15 minutes **Baking Time:** 20 minutes
Total Time: 35 minutes

Ingredients:

- 2 medium zucchinis, thinly sliced
- 2 tablespoons olive oil
- $^1/_2$ cup breadcrumbs (preferably whole wheat)
- $^1/_4$ cup grated Parmesan cheese
- 1 teaspoon garlic powder
- 1 teaspoon dried oregano
- $^1/_2$ teaspoon salt
- $^1/_4$ teaspoon black pepper
- Cooking spray (olive oil or non-stick)

Instructions:

1. Preheat the oven to 425°F (220°C).
2. In a bowl, combine sliced zucchinis with olive oil and toss until evenly coated.
3. In a separate bowl, mix breadcrumbs, Parmesan cheese, garlic powder, oregano, salt, and black pepper.
4. Dip each zucchini slice into the breadcrumb mixture, pressing gently to adhere the coating.
5. Place the coated zucchini slices on a baking sheet lined with parchment paper and lightly sprayed with cooking spray.

6. Bake in the preheated oven for 18-20 minutes or until the zucchini chips are golden and crispy.
7. Remove from the oven and let them cool for a few minutes.
8. Serve the Baked Zucchini Chips as a healthy and satisfying snack.

Simple Edamame Recipe:

Servings: 4 **Preparation Time**: 5 minutes **Cooking Time**: 5 minutes **Total Time**: 10 minutes

---

Ingredients:

- 2 cups frozen edamame in the pods
- 1 tablespoon sea salt (for boiling)
- **Optional:** Sesame seeds, soy sauce, or chili flakes for seasoning

Instructions:

1. Bring a pot of water to a boil and add sea salt.
2. Add the frozen edamame pods to the boiling water.
3. Cook for approximately 5 minutes or until the edamame is tender.
4. Drain the edamame and transfer them to a bowl.
5. Optionally, sprinkle sesame seeds, drizzle with soy sauce, or add chili flakes for extra flavor.
6. Toss the edamame gently to coat with the seasoning.
7. Serve the Simple Edamame warm and enjoy it as a nutritious and tasty snack.

Caprese Skewers Recipe:

Servings: 4 (makes about 16 skewers) **Preparation Time:** 15 minutes
Assembly Time: 10 minutes **Total Time:** 25 minutes

Ingredients:

- 1 pint cherry tomatoes
- 1 pound fresh mozzarella, cut into bite-sized pieces.Fresh basil leaves
- Balsamic glaze for drizzling
- Extra virgin olive oil for drizzling
- Salt and black pepper to taste
- Wooden skewers

Instructions:

1. Wash the cherry tomatoes and basil leaves.
2. On each skewer, thread a cherry tomato, a piece of fresh mozzarella, and a basil leaf.
3. Repeat the process until each skewer is filled.
4. Arrange the Caprese Skewers on a serving platter.
5. Drizzle balsamic glaze and extra virgin olive oil over the skewers.
6. Sprinkle it with salt and black pepper to taste.
7. Serve immediately and enjoy this elegant and delicious appetizer.

Roasted Chickpeas Recipe:

Servings: 4 **Preparation Time:** 10 minutes **Baking Time:** 25-30 minutes **Total Time:** 40 minutes

---

Ingredients:

- 2 cans (15 oz each) chickpeas, drained and rinsed
- 2 tablespoons olive oil
- 1 teaspoon ground cumin
- 1 teaspoon smoked paprika
- $^1/_2$ teaspoon garlic powder
- $^1/_2$ teaspoon onion powder
- $^1/_2$ teaspoon cayenne pepper (adjust to taste)
- Salt and black pepper to taste

Instructions:

1. Preheat the oven to 400°F (200°C).
2. Pat dry the rinsed chickpeas with a paper towel to remove excess moisture.
3. In a bowl, toss the chickpeas with olive oil, cumin, smoked paprika, garlic powder, onion powder, cayenne pepper, salt, and black pepper.
4. Spread the seasoned chickpeas in a single layer on a baking sheet lined with parchment paper.
5. Roast in the preheated oven for 25-30 minutes, or until the chickpeas are crispy and golden brown.
6. Shake the baking sheet halfway through the cooking time for even roasting.
7. Remove from the oven and let the Roasted Chickpeas cool for a few minutes before serving.
8. Enjoy these crunchy and flavorful Roasted Chickpeas as a snack or salad topper.

8

SIDE DISHES

Brown Rice Pilaf

Serving: 4 **Preparation Time:** 10 minutes **Cooking Time:** 45 minutes
Total Time: 55 minutes

Ingredients:

- 1 cup brown rice
- 2 tablespoons olive oil or butter
- $^1/_2$ onion, finely chopped
- 2 cloves garlic, minced
- 1 carrot, diced
- 1 celery stalk, diced
- $^1/_4$ cup slivered almonds (optional, for added crunch)
- 2 cups vegetable or chicken broth
- 1 teaspoon dried thyme
- Salt and pepper to taste
- Fresh parsley, chopped (for garnish)

Instructions:

1. Rinse the brown rice under cold water until the water runs clear.
2. In a large skillet or saucepan, heat olive oil or butter over medium heat.
3. Add chopped onion and sauté until softened, about 3-5 minutes.
4. Add minced garlic, diced carrot, and diced celery. Sauté for an additional 3-5 minutes.

5. Stir in slivered almonds (if using) and continue cooking for 2 minutes until they are lightly toasted.
6. Add brown rice to the skillet and cook, stirring frequently, for another 2 minutes to toast the rice.
7. Pour in vegetable or chicken broth. Add dried thyme, salt, and pepper to taste. Bring to a boil.
8. Reduce the heat to low, cover the skillet, and simmer for 40-45 minutes or until the rice is tender and the liquid is absorbed.
9. Once cooked, fluff the rice with a fork.
10.   Garnish with chopped fresh parsley before serving.

Roasted Brussels Sprouts

Serving: 4 **Preparation Time:** 10 minutes **Roasting Time:** 25-30 minutes **Total Time:** 35-40 minutes

Ingredients:

- 1 lb (450g) Brussels sprouts, trimmed and halved
- 2 tablespoons olive oil
- Salt and pepper to taste
- Optional: 1-2 tablespoons balsamic vinegar or grated Parmesan cheese for added flavor

Instructions:

1. Preheat the oven to 400°F (200°C).
2. In a large bowl, toss Brussels sprouts with olive oil, ensuring they are evenly coated.

3. Spread the Brussels sprouts in a single layer on a baking sheet.
4. Season with salt and pepper to taste.
5. Roast in the preheated oven for 25-30 minutes or until the Brussels sprouts are golden brown and crisp on the edges, with a tender interior.
6. Optional: If desired, drizzle balsamic vinegar over the roasted Brussels sprouts for a tangy flavor or sprinkle grated Parmesan cheese for added richness.
7. Remove from the oven and serve immediately.

Quinoa-Stuffed Bell Peppers

Serving: 4 **Preparation Time:** 15 minutes **Cooking Time:** 30 minutes
Total Time: 45 minutes

Ingredients:

- 4 bell peppers, halved and seeds removed
- 1 cup quinoa, rinsed
- 2 cups vegetable broth
- 1 tablespoon olive oil
- 1 onion, finely chopped
- 2 cloves garlic, minced
- 1 zucchini, diced
- 1 carrot, grated
- 1 cup black beans, drained and rinsed
- 1 cup corn kernels (fresh or frozen)
- 1 teaspoon ground cumin
- 1 teaspoon smoked paprika
- Salt and pepper to taste

- 1 cup tomato sauce
- 1 cup shredded cheese (cheddar or Mexican blend)
- Fresh cilantro or parsley for garnish

Instructions:

1. Preheat the oven to 375°F (190°C).
2. Place the halved bell peppers in a baking dish.
3. In a saucepan, combine quinoa and vegetable broth. Bring to a boil, then reduce heat, cover, and simmer for 15-20 minutes or until quinoa is cooked and liquid is absorbed.
4. In a large skillet, heat olive oil over medium heat. Add chopped onion and garlic, sauté until softened.
5. Add diced zucchini, grated carrot, black beans, and corn to the skillet. Cook for an additional 5 minutes.
6. Stir in cooked quinoa, ground cumin, smoked paprika, salt, and pepper. Mix well.
7. Fill each bell pepper half with the quinoa mixture.
8. Spoon tomato sauce over each stuffed pepper.
9. Sprinkle shredded cheese on top.
10. Cover the baking dish with foil and bake in the preheated oven for 20 minutes. Remove the foil and bake for an additional 10 minutes or until the cheese is melted and bubbly.
11. Garnish with fresh cilantro or parsley before serving.

Farro and Vegetable Pilaf

Serving: 4 **Preparation Time:** 10 minutes **Cooking Time:** 30-35 minutes **Total Time:** 40-45 minutes

Ingredients:

- 1 cup farro, rinsed and drained
- 2 tablespoons olive oil
- 1 onion, finely chopped
- 2 cloves garlic, minced
- 1 carrot, diced
- 1 zucchini, diced
- 1 red bell pepper, diced
- 1 cup cherry tomatoes, halved
- 2 cups vegetable broth
- 1 teaspoon dried thyme
- Salt and pepper to taste
- $^1/_4$ cup fresh parsley, chopped (for garnish)
- Grated Parmesan cheese (optional, for serving)

Instructions:

1. In a medium saucepan, heat olive oil over medium heat. Add chopped onion and sauté until softened.
2. Add minced garlic and cook for an additional 1-2 minutes.
3. Stir in farro and cook for 2-3 minutes to lightly toast the grains.
4. Add diced carrot, zucchini, red bell pepper, and cherry tomatoes. Cook for another 3-5 minutes.
5. Pour in vegetable broth, add dried thyme, and season with salt and pepper to taste. Bring to a boil.
6. Reduce the heat to low, cover the saucepan, and simmer for 25-30 minutes or until the farro is tender and the liquid is absorbed.
7. Remove from heat and let the pilaf sit, covered, for 5 minutes.
8. Fluff the farro and vegetable mixture with a fork.
9. Garnish with chopped fresh parsley and, if desired, serve with grated Parmesan cheese.

Baked Zucchini Fries

Serving: 4 **Preparation Time:** 15 minutes **Cooking Time:** 20 minutes
Total Time: 35 minutes

Ingredients:

- 2 medium zucchinis, cut into fries
- 1 cup whole wheat breadcrumbs
- $1/2$ cup grated Parmesan cheese
- 1 teaspoon dried oregano
- 1 teaspoon garlic powder
- $1/2$ teaspoon paprika
- Salt and pepper to taste
- 2 eggs, beaten
- Olive oil cooking spray

Instructions:

1. Preheat the oven to 425°F (220°C). Line a baking sheet with parchment paper.
2. In a shallow bowl, mix whole wheat breadcrumbs, grated Parmesan cheese, dried oregano, garlic powder, paprika, salt, and pepper.
3. Dip each zucchini fry into the beaten eggs, ensuring it's well-coated.
4. Roll the coated zucchini fry in the breadcrumb mixture, pressing gently to adhere the crumbs.
5. Place the coated zucchini fries on the prepared baking sheet, leaving space between each fry.
6. Lightly spray the zucchini fries with olive oil cooking spray.
7. Bake in the preheated oven for about 18-20 minutes or until the zucchini fries are golden brown and crispy.
8. Serve immediately with your favorite dipping sauce, such as marinara or tzatziki.

Garlic Roasted Sweet Potatoes

Serving: 4 **Preparation Time:** 15 minutes **Cooking Time:** 25 minutes **Total Time:** 40 minutes

---

Ingredients:

- 3 medium sweet potatoes, peeled and cut into cubes
- 3 tablespoons olive oil
- 4 cloves garlic, minced
- 1 teaspoon dried rosemary (or 1 tablespoon fresh rosemary, chopped)
- Salt and pepper to taste
- Fresh parsley for garnish (optional)

Instructions:

1. Preheat the oven to 425°F (220°C). Line a baking sheet with parchment paper.
2. In a large bowl, toss sweet potato cubes with olive oil, minced garlic, dried rosemary, salt, and pepper until evenly coated.
3. Spread the sweet potato mixture in a single layer on the prepared baking sheet.
4. Roast in the preheated oven for about 25-30 minutes, or until the sweet potatoes are tender and have a golden-brown crust, tossing halfway through for even cooking.
5. Once roasted, remove from the oven and garnish with fresh parsley if desired.
6. Serve the Garlic Roasted Sweet Potatoes as a flavorful and nutritious side dish.

These roasted sweet potatoes are a delicious and aromatic addition to your meal, providing a balance of sweet and savory flavors. Enjoy!

Mashed Cauliflower with Chives

Serving: 4 **Preparation Time:** 15 minutes **Cooking Time:** 15 minutes **Total Time:** 30 minutes

---

Ingredients:

- 1 large head of cauliflower, cut into florets
- 2 cloves garlic, minced
- 2 tablespoons unsalted butter or olive oil
- $\frac{1}{4}$ cup plain Greek yogurt
- Salt and pepper to taste
- 2 tablespoons fresh chives, chopped

Instructions:

1. Steam or boil the cauliflower florets until they are tender, about 10-12 minutes.
2. Drain the cauliflower and transfer it to a large bowl.
3. Using a potato masher or a food processor, mash the cauliflower until it reaches a smooth consistency.
4. In a small pan, sauté minced garlic in butter or olive oil until fragrant.
5. Add the sautéed garlic, Greek yogurt, salt, and pepper to the mashed cauliflower. Continue mashing or blending until well combined.
6. Adjust salt and pepper to taste, and fold in chopped chives.
7. Serve the Mashed Cauliflower with Chives as a creamy and flavorful alternative to traditional mashed potatoes.

This dish is a low-carb and nutritious option that pairs well with various proteins or can stand alone as a tasty side. Enjoy!

Grilled Asparagus with Parmesan

Serving: 4 **Preparation Time:** 10 minutes **Cooking Time:** 8 minutes
Total Time: 18 minutes

Ingredients:

1 bunch of fresh asparagus spears, tough ends trimmed
2 tablespoons olive oil
Salt and pepper to taste
$^{1}/_{4}$ cup grated Parmesan cheese
Lemon wedges for serving (optional)

Instructions:

1. Preheat the grill to medium-high heat.
2. In a large bowl, toss asparagus spears with olive oil, salt, and pepper until evenly coated.
3. Place the asparagus on the preheated grill grates, arranging them in a single layer.
4. Grill for about 3-4 minutes per side, or until the asparagus is tender and has grill marks.
5. Remove the grilled asparagus from the heat and transfer to a serving platter.
6. Sprinkle grated Parmesan cheese over the hot asparagus, allowing it to melt slightly.
7. **Optional:** Squeeze lemon wedges over the asparagus for a fresh citrusy flavor.

8. Serve the Grilled Asparagus with Parmesan as a delicious and nutritious side dish.

This dish is a perfect combination of smoky grilled asparagus and the savory richness of Parmesan cheese. Enjoy!

Green Bean Almondine

Serving: 4 **Preparation Time:** 10 minutes **Cooking Time:** 10 minutes **Total Time:** 20 minutes

---

Ingredients:

- 1 pound fresh green beans, trimmed
- 2 tablespoons unsalted butter
- 2 tablespoons olive oil
- 1/3 cup slivered almonds
- 2 cloves garlic, minced
- 1 tablespoon lemon juice
- Salt and pepper to taste
- Fresh parsley for garnish (optional)

Instructions:

1. Bring a large pot of salted water to a boil. Add green beans and cook for about 2-3 minutes, or until they are bright green and slightly tender. Drain and set aside.

2. In a large skillet, heat butter and olive oil over medium heat.
3. Add slivered almonds to the skillet and sauté for 2-3 minutes, or until they are lightly toasted.
4. Stir in minced garlic and cook for an additional 1-2 minutes until fragrant.
5. Add the blanched green beans to the skillet and toss to coat them in the almond and garlic mixture.
6. Drizzle lemon juice over the green beans and continue tossing until the beans are well coated.
7. Season with salt and pepper to taste.
8. **Optional:** Garnish with fresh parsley before serving.

Roasted Brussels Sprouts with Garlic:

Serving: 4 **Preparation Time:** 10 minutes **Cooking Time:** 20-25 minutes **Total Time:** 30-35 minutes

Ingredients:

- Brussels sprouts, trimmed and halved
- Olive oil
- Minced garlic
- Salt and pepper to taste

Instructions:

1. Preheat your oven to 400°F (200°C).
2. In a bowl, toss the halved Brussels sprouts with olive oil, minced garlic, salt, and pepper. Ensure the Brussels sprouts are evenly coated.
3. Spread the Brussels sprouts on a baking sheet in a single layer.
4. Season with salt and pepper to taste

5. Roast in the preheated oven for about 20-25 minutes or until they are golden brown and crispy on the edges. Stir halfway through to ensure even cooking.

6. **Optional:** If desired, drizzle balsamic vinegar over the roasted Brussels sprouts for a tangy flavor or sprinkle grated Parmesan cheese for added richness.

7. Remove from the oven and serve immediately.

9

DESSERTS

Dark Chocolate-Dipped Strawberries

Serving: Varies (depending on the quantity of strawberries)
Preparation Time: 15 minutes **Chilling Time:** 30 minutes **Total Time:** 45 minutes

Ingredients:

- Fresh strawberries, washed and dried
- 4 ounces (about 120g) dark chocolate, chopped
- 1 teaspoon coconut oil or vegetable oil (optional, for smoother chocolate)
- Toppings of choice: chopped nuts, shredded coconut, or sea salt

Instructions:

1. Line a baking sheet with parchment paper.
2. In a heatproof bowl, melt the dark chocolate in the microwave or using a double boiler. If using a microwave, heat in 20-second intervals, stirring between each interval until fully melted.
3. If desired, add coconut oil or vegetable oil to the melted chocolate for a smoother consistency. Stir well to combine.
4. Hold each strawberry by the stem and dip it into the melted chocolate, ensuring the strawberry is fully coated.
5. Allow excess chocolate to drip off, then place the dipped strawberry on the prepared baking sheet.

6. Quickly sprinkle the dipped strawberry with your choice of toppings while the chocolate is still wet.
7. Repeat the dipping process for each strawberry.
8. Place the baking sheet in the refrigerator for at least 30 minutes or until the chocolate hardens.
9. Once the chocolate is set, transfer the dark chocolate- dipped strawberries to a serving plate
10. Serve and enjoy these delightful treats!

Dark Chocolate-Dipped Strawberries are a decadent yet relatively healthy dessert option, combining the sweetness of ripe strawberries with the richness of dark chocolate. Enjoy in moderation!

Berry and Yogurt Parfait

Serving: 2 **Preparation Time:** 10 minutes **Total Time:** 10 minutes

Ingredients:

- 1 cup Greek yogurt
- 1 cup mixed berries (strawberries, blueberries, raspberries)
- $^1/_2$ cup granola
- 1 tablespoon honey or maple syrup (optional, for drizzling)
- Fresh mint leaves (optional, for garnish)

Instructions:

1. In serving glasses or bowls, start by layering a spoonful of Greek yogurt at the bottom.
2. Add a layer of mixed berries on top of the yogurt.
3. Sprinkle a layer of granola over the berries.

4. Repeat the layers until the glasses are filled, finishing with a final layer of berries and granola on top.
5. Optionally, drizzle honey or maple syrup over the parfait for added sweetness.
6. Garnish with fresh mint leaves if desired.
7. Serve the Berry and Yogurt Parfait immediately and enjoy this delightful and nutritious treat!

Fruit Sorbet

Serving: 4 **Preparation Time:** 10 minutes **Freezing Time:** 4-6 hours
Total Time: 4-6 hours and 10 minutes

Ingredients:

- 3 cups mixed fresh or frozen fruits (e.g., berries, mango, pineapple)
- $^1/_2$ cup granulated sugar
- $^1/_4$ cup water
- 1 tablespoon fresh lemon or lime juice

Instructions:

1. In a small saucepan, combine sugar and water. Heat over medium heat, stirring occasionally, until the sugar is completely dissolved. Allow the simple syrup to cool.
2. Place the mixed fruits in a blender or food processor.
3. Add the cooled simple syrup and fresh lemon or lime juice to the blender with the fruits.
4. Blend until the mixture is smooth and well combined.
5. Strain the fruit mixture through a fine-mesh sieve to remove any seeds or solids if desired.

6. Pour the sorbet mixture into a shallow dish, cover, and place it in the freezer.
7. Every 30 minutes for the first 2-3 hours, use a fork to stir and break up any ice crystals that form.
8. Continue freezing for 4-6 hours or until the sorbet reaches a firm, scoopable consistency.
9. Before serving, let the sorbet sit at room temperature for a few minutes to soften slightly.
10. Scoop the Fruit Sorbet into bowls or cones and enjoy this refreshing and naturally sweetened dessert!

Apple Cinnamon Oat Bars

Yield: 12 bars **Preparation Time:** 15 minutes **Baking Time:** 25-30 minutes **Cooling Time:** 1 hour **Total Time:** 1 hour and 45 minutes

Ingredients:

- 2 cups old-fashioned oats
- 1 cup all-purpose flour
- $1/2$ cup brown sugar, packed
- $1/2$ teaspoon baking soda
- $1/4$ teaspoon salt
- 1 teaspoon ground cinnamon
- $1/2$ cup unsalted butter, melted
- 1 large egg
- 1 teaspoon vanilla extract
- 2 cups apples, peeled and diced
- 1 tablespoon lemon juice
- 2 tablespoons granulated sugar (for sprinkling)

Instructions:

1. Preheat the oven to 350°F (175°C). Grease or line a 9x9-inch (23x23 cm) baking pan with parchment paper.
2. In a large bowl, combine oats, all-purpose flour, brown sugar, baking soda, salt, and ground cinnamon.
3. In a separate bowl, whisk together melted butter, egg, and vanilla extract.
4. Add the wet ingredients to the dry ingredients, stirring until well combined.
5. In a medium bowl, toss diced apples with lemon juice and granulated sugar.
6. Fold the diced apples into the oat mixture until evenly distributed.
7. Press the mixture into the prepared baking pan, spreading it out evenly.
8. Optionally, sprinkle an additional tablespoon of granulated sugar over the top for a slightly crunchy texture.
9. Bake in the preheated oven for 25-30 minutes or until the edges are golden brown and a toothpick inserted into the center comes out clean.
10. Allow the Apple Cinnamon Oat Bars to cool in the pan for 10 minutes before transferring them to a wire rack to cool completely.
11. Once cooled, cut into bars and enjoy these delicious and wholesome Apple Cinnamon Oat Bars!

Cinnamon Baked Pears

Serving: 4 **Preparation Time:** 10 minutes **Baking Time:** 25 minutes **Total Time:** 35 minutes

Ingredients:

- 4 ripe pears, halved and cored
- 2 tablespoons melted unsalted butter or coconut oil
- 2 tablespoons honey or maple syrup
- 1 teaspoon ground cinnamon
- $^1/_4$ teaspoon ground nutmeg
- **Optional:** Chopped nuts for garnish
- **Optional:** Greek yogurt or vanilla ice cream for serving

Instructions:

1. Preheat the oven to 375°F (190°C). Grease a baking dish.
2. Place the pear halves, cut side up, in the prepared baking dish.
3. In a small bowl, whisk together melted butter (or coconut oil), honey (or maple syrup), ground cinnamon, and ground nutmeg.
4. Brush the cinnamon mixture over the top of each pear half, ensuring they are well-coated.
5. Bake in the preheated oven for about 25 minutes, or until the pears are tender and slightly caramelized.
6. **Optional:** During the last 5 minutes of baking, sprinkle chopped nuts over the pears for added crunch.
7. Remove the baked pears from the oven and let them cool slightly.
8. Serve the Cinnamon Baked Pears warm, either on their own or with a dollop of Greek yogurt or a scoop of vanilla ice cream.

These Cinnamon Baked Pears are a simple yet elegant dessert, highlighting the natural sweetness of the pears with warm cinnamon flavors. Enjoy!

Oatmeal Raisin Cookies

Yield: Approximately 24 cookies **Preparation Time:** 15 minutes
Baking Time: 10-12 minutes **Total Time:** 25-27 minutes

Ingredients:

- 1 cup old-fashioned oats
- $^3/_4$ cup whole wheat flour
- $^1/_2$ teaspoon baking soda
- $^1/_2$ teaspoon ground cinnamon
- $^1/_2$ teaspoon salt
- $^1/_2$ cup unsalted butter, softened
- $^1/_2$ cup coconut sugar or brown sugar
- 1 large egg
- 1 teaspoon vanilla extract
- $^1/_2$ cup raisins

Instructions:

1. Preheat the oven to 350°F (175°C). Line a baking sheet with parchment paper.
2. In a medium bowl, combine oats, whole wheat flour, baking soda, ground cinnamon, and salt. Set aside.
3. In a large bowl, cream together softened butter and coconut sugar (or brown sugar) until light and fluffy.
4. Beat in the egg and vanilla extract until well combined.
5. Gradually add the dry ingredients to the wet ingredients, mixing until just combined.
6. Fold in the raisins until evenly distributed throughout the cookie dough.
7. Drop rounded tablespoons of dough onto the prepared baking sheet, spacing them about 2 inches apart.

8. Bake in the preheated oven for 10-12 minutes or until the edges are golden brown.
9. Allow the cookies to cool on the baking sheet for a few minutes before transferring them to a wire rack to cool completely.

Baked Blueberry Oat Bars

Yield: 12 bars **Preparation Time:** 15 minutes **Baking Time:** 30-35 minutes **Total Time:** 45-50 minutes

---

Ingredients:

- 2 cups old-fashioned oats
- 1 cup whole wheat flour
- $\frac{1}{2}$ cup coconut sugar or brown sugar
- $\frac{1}{2}$ teaspoon baking powder
- $\frac{1}{2}$ teaspoon salt
- $\frac{1}{2}$ cup unsalted butter, melted
- 1 large egg, beaten
- 1 teaspoon vanilla extract
- 1 cup fresh or frozen blueberries

Instructions:

1. Preheat the oven to 350°F (175°C). Grease or line a square baking dish (8x8 inches or similar) with parchment paper.
2. In a large bowl, combine oats, whole wheat flour, coconut sugar (or brown sugar), baking powder, and salt.
3. In a separate bowl, whisk together melted butter, beaten egg, and vanilla extract.

4. Pour the wet ingredients into the dry ingredients and mix until well combined.
5. Gently fold in the blueberries, ensuring they are evenly distributed in the mixture.
6. Press the mixture evenly into the prepared baking dish.
7. Bake in the preheated oven for 30-35 minutes or until the edges are golden brown and a toothpick inserted into the center comes out clean.
8. Allow the bars to cool in the baking dish for at least 10 minutes before transferring them to a wire rack to cool completely.
9. Once cooled, cut into bars and serve.

Watermelon Mint Salad

Serving: 4 **Preparation Time:** 15 minutes **Total Time:** 15 minutes

Ingredients:

- 4 cups seedless watermelon, diced
- $^1/_2$ cup fresh mint leaves, finely chopped
- 1 tablespoon honey or maple syrup
- 1 tablespoon fresh lime juice
- **Optional:** Feta cheese, crumbled (for added flavor)

Instructions:

1. In a large bowl, combine diced watermelon and chopped mint.
2. In a small bowl, whisk together honey or maple syrup and fresh lime juice to create the dressing.
3. Drizzle the dressing over the watermelon and mint mixture, tossing gently to coat evenly.

4. If desired, sprinkle crumbled feta cheese over the salad for an extra layer of flavor.
5. Serve the Watermelon Mint Salad immediately, or refrigerate for a short time to enhance the refreshing chill.

Cinnamon Baked Pears

Serving: 4 **Preparation Time:** 10 minutes **Baking Time:** 25 minutes **Total Time:** 35 minutes

---

Ingredients:

- 4 ripe pears, halved and cored
- 2 tablespoons melted unsalted butter or coconut oil
- 2 tablespoons honey or maple syrup
- 1 teaspoon ground cinnamon
- $1/_2$ teaspoon ground nutmeg
- **Optional:** Chopped nuts for garnish
- **Optional:** Greek yogurt or vanilla ice cream for serving

Instructions:

1. Preheat the oven to 375°F (190°C). Grease a baking dish.
2. Place the pear halves, cut side up, in the prepared baking dish.
3. In a small bowl, whisk together melted butter (or coconut oil), honey (or maple syrup), ground cinnamon, and ground nutmeg.
4. Brush the cinnamon mixture over the top of each pear half, ensuring they are well-coated.
5. Bake in the preheated oven for about 25 minutes, or until the pears are tender and slightly caramelized.

6. **Optional:** During the last 5 minutes of baking, sprinkle chopped nuts over the pears for added crunch.
7. Remove the baked pears from the oven and let them cool slightly.
8. Serve the Cinnamon Baked Pears warm, either on their own or with a dollop of Greek yogurt or a scoop of vanilla ice cream.

Baked Blueberry Oat Bars

Yield: Approximately 12 bars **Preparation Time:** 15 minutes **Baking Time:** 30-35 minutes **Total Time:** 45-50 minutes

Ingredients:

- 2 cups old-fashioned oats
- 1 cup whole wheat flour
- $1/2$ cup coconut sugar or brown sugar
- $1/2$ teaspoon baking powder
- $1/4$ teaspoon salt
- $1/2$ cup unsalted butter, melted
- 1 large egg, beaten
- 1 teaspoon vanilla extract
- 1 cup fresh or frozen blueberries

Instructions:

1. Preheat the oven to 350°F (175°C). Grease or line a square baking dish (8x8 inches or similar) with parchment paper.
2. In a large bowl, combine oats, whole wheat flour, coconut sugar (or brown sugar), baking powder, and salt.
3. In a separate bowl, whisk together melted butter, beaten egg, and vanilla extract.

4. Pour the wet ingredients into the dry ingredients and mix until well combined.
5. Gently fold in the blueberries, ensuring they are evenly distributed in the mixture.
6. Press the mixture evenly into the prepared baking dish.
7. Bake in the preheated oven for 30-35 minutes or until the edges are golden brown and a toothpick inserted into the center comes out clean.
8. Allow the bars to cool in the baking dish for at least 10 minutes before transferring them to a wire rack to cool completely.
9. Once cooled, cut into bars and serve.

10

BEVERAGES

Infused Water Varieties

Citrus Mint Infused Water

Ingredients:

- Slices of lemon, lime, and orange
- Fresh mint leaves
- Ice cubes

Instructions: Combine citrus slices and mint leaves in a pitcher, add ice cubes, fill with water, and let it infuse in the refrigerator for a refreshing drink.

Berry Basil Infused Water

Ingredients:

- Mixed berries (strawberries, blueberries, raspberries)
- Fresh basil leaves
- Ice cubes

Instructions: Mix berries and basil in a pitcher, add ice cubes, fill with water, and let it infuse for a burst of fruity flavor.

Cucumber Rosemary Infused Water

Ingredients:

- Sliced cucumber
- Fresh rosemary sprigs
- Ice cubes

Instructions: Combine cucumber slices and rosemary in a pitcher, add ice cubes, fill with water, and let it infuse for a crisp and herbal-infused water.

Pineapple Coconut Infused Water

Ingredients:

- Pineapple chunks
- Coconut water
- Ice cubes

Instructions: Combine pineapple chunks with coconut water in a pitcher, add ice cubes, let it chill in the refrigerator, and enjoy a tropical twist.

Watermelon Basil Infused Water

Ingredients:

- Watermelon cubes
- Fresh basil leaves
- Ice cubes

Instructions: Mix watermelon cubes and basil in a pitcher, add ice cubes, fill with water, and let it infuse for a sweet and aromatic watermelon treat.

Ginger Lemon Infused Water

Ingredients:

- Sliced ginger
- Lemon slices
- Ice cubes

Instructions: Combine sliced ginger and lemon in a pitcher, add ice cubes, fill with water, and let it infuse for a zesty and invigorating drink.

Fresh Fruit Juice Blends

Citrus Berry Blast

Ingredients:

- Oranges (peeled and segmented)
- Strawberries (hulled)
- Blueberries
- Pineapple chunks

Instructions: Run the fruits through a juicer or blender, mix the juices, and enjoy this zesty and antioxidant-rich blend.

Tropical Paradise

Ingredients:

- Mango chunks
- Pineapple slices
- Kiwi (peeled and sliced)
- Coconut water

Instructions: Juice or blend the tropical fruits, mix with coconut water, and savor the taste of the tropics.

Berry Citrus Medley

Ingredients:

- Raspberries
- Blackberries
- Grapefruit (peeled and segmented)
- Lime (peeled)

Instructions: Juice or blend the berries with grapefruit and lime for a refreshing and tangy medley.

Watermelon Mint Splash

Ingredients:

- Watermelon cubes (seedless)
- Fresh mint leaves
- Lime (peeled)

Instructions: Juice or blend watermelon with mint and lime for a hydrating and minty watermelon splash.

Apple Ginger Zing

Ingredients:

- Apples (cored and sliced)

- Fresh ginger (peeled)
- Lemon (peeled)

Instructions: Juice or blend apples with ginger and lemon for a zesty and invigorating apple ginger zing.

Pineapple Basil Breeze

Ingredients:

- Pineapple chunks
- Fresh basil leaves
- Green apple (cored and sliced)

Instructions: Juice or blend pineapple with basil and green apple for a tropical and herbal-infused breeze.

Vegetable Smoothie Recipe:

Preparation Time: 5 minutes **Total Time:** 5 minutes

Ingredients:

- 1 cup spinach
- 1 cup kale
- $\frac{1}{2}$ cucumber, peeled and sliced
- 1 medium carrot, peeled and chopped
- 1 cup water or low fat yogurt
- **Optional:** honey or lemon for added flavor

Instructions:

1. Wash and prepare the vegetables by chopping them into smaller pieces for easier blending.

2. In a blender, combine spinach, kale, cucumber, carrot, and water (or low fat yogurt).
3. Blend on high speed until the mixture is smooth and well combined. Adjust the thickness by adding more water or yogurt if needed.
4. Taste the smoothie and add honey or a squeeze of lemon for extra flavor, if desired.
5. Pour the vegetable smoothie into a glass and enjoy it as a nutritious and refreshing beverage.

Cranberry Sparkle Recipe:

Total Time: 5 minutes **Preparation Time:** 5 minutes

Ingredients:

- 1 cup cranberry juice
- $\frac{1}{2}$ cup sparkling water
- Ice cubes
- 1 lime, sliced for garnish

Instructions:

1. In a glass, combine cranberry juice and sparkling water.
2. Stir well to mix the liquids.
3. Add ice cubes to the glass to chill the drink.
4. Garnish with slices of lime for a citrusy twist.
5. Stir again before enjoying your Cranberry Sparkle.

Orange Carrot Juice:

Serving: 2 servings **Preparation Time:** 10 minutes

Ingredients:

- 4 large carrots, peeled and chopped
- 3 large oranges, peeled and segmented
- 1 tablespoon fresh ginger, grated (optional for added flavor)

Instructions:

1. In a juicer, combine the chopped carrots, segmented oranges, and grated ginger (if using).
2. Process the ingredients through the juicer according to its instructions.
3. Once juiced, stir the mixture to combine flavors.
4. Pour the juice into glasses.
5. Optionally, chill the juice in the refrigerator before serving.

Lemon Ginger Detox Water Recipe:

Servings: 1 **Preparation Time:** 5 minutes **Total Time:** 5 minutes

---

Ingredients:

- 1 lemon, thinly sliced
- 1 inch piece of fresh ginger, peeled and sliced
- 2 cups water
- Ice cubes (optional)
- Fresh mint leaves for garnish (optional)

Instructions:

1. In a pitcher or large glass, combine the thinly sliced lemon and peeled, sliced ginger.
2. Pour 2 cups of water over the lemon and ginger.
3. If you prefer a chilled drink, add ice cubes to the water.
4. Stir the mixture gently to infuse the flavors.
5. Let the Lemon Ginger Detox Water sit for a few minutes to allow the flavors to meld.
6. Optionally, garnish with fresh mint leaves for added freshness.
7. Sip and enjoy this refreshing and detoxifying beverage.

Hibiscus Iced Tea Recipe:

Servings: 4 **Preparation Time:** 5 minutes **Total Time:** 10 minutes (plus cooling time)

Ingredients:

- 4 hibiscus tea bags
- 4 cups boiling water
- 23 tablespoons honey (adjust to taste)
- Ice cubes
- Orange slices or mint leaves for garnish (optional)

Instructions:

1. Place hibiscus tea bags in a heat proof pitcher.
2. Pour boiling water over the tea bags and let steep for 5 minutes.
3. Remove the tea bags and stir in honey until it dissolves.
4. Allow the tea to cool to room temperature, then refrigerate until chilled.
5. Once chilled, serve the Hibiscus Iced Tea over ice cubes.
6. Garnish with orange slices or mint leaves if desired.
7. Stir and enjoy this vibrant and refreshing iced tea.

11

MEALS PLANS

7-Day DASH Diet Meal Plan

Day 1:

Breakfast: Greek yogurt with mixed berries and a sprinkle of almonds.
Lunch: Grilled chicken salad with mixed greens, cherry tomatoes, cucumbers, and olive oil vinaigrette.
Snack: Carrot sticks with hummus.
Dinner: Baked salmon with quinoa and steamed broccoli.

Day 2:

Breakfast: Oatmeal with sliced banana and a drizzle of honey.
Lunch: Quinoa salad with chickpeas, cherry tomatoes, bell peppers, and a lemon-tahini dressing.
Snack: Apple slices with a small portion of low-fat cheese.
Dinner: Turkey and vegetable stir-fry with brown rice.

Day 3:

Breakfast: Whole grain toast with avocado and poached eggs.
Lunch: Lentil soup with a side of mixed green salad.
Snack: Greek yogurt with a handful of walnuts.
Dinner: Baked cod with tomato basil salsa, sweet potato wedges, and asparagus.

Day 4:

Breakfast: Smoothie bowl with spinach, banana, berries, and a sprinkle of chia seeds.
Lunch: Chickpea and spinach curry with brown rice.
Snack: Fresh fruit salad.
Dinner: Grilled chicken breast with roasted vegetables (zucchini, bell peppers, and carrots).

Day 5:

Breakfast: Cottage cheese with sliced peaches and a drizzle of honey.
Lunch: Spaghetti squash primavera with tomato sauce and a side of mixed greens.
Snack: Celery sticks with peanut butter.
Dinner: Teriyaki tofu stir-fry with quinoa and broccoli.

Day 6:

Breakfast: Scrambled eggs with sautéed spinach and whole grain toast.
Lunch: Quinoa-stuffed bell peppers with a side of mixed greens.
Snack: Mixed nuts (almonds, walnuts, and pistachios).
Dinner: Baked salmon with lemon and herbs, sweet potato mash, and green beans.

Day 7:

Breakfast: Whole grain waffles with fresh berries and a dollop of Greek yogurt.
Lunch: Lentil salad with mixed vegetables, feta cheese, and balsamic vinaigrette.
Snack: Orange slices with a handful of almonds.
Dinner: Grilled shrimp skewers with quinoa and roasted Brussels sprouts.

Remember to stay hydrated with water or herbal teas throughout the day. Adjust portion sizes based on individual needs and consult with a healthcare professional or a registered dietitian before making significant changes to your diet.

Quick and Easy Weeknight Dinners

1. One-Pan Chicken and Vegetables:

- Season chicken breasts with your favorite spices.
- Place them on a baking sheet with a mix of chopped vegetables (e.g., bell peppers, zucchini, cherry tomatoes).
- Drizzle with olive oil, bake until the chicken is cooked through, and veggies are tender.

2. Stir-Fried Shrimp with Broccoli:

- Stir-fry shrimp with broccoli, bell peppers, and snap peas in a wok.
- Add soy sauce, garlic, and ginger for flavor.

Serve over brown rice or noodles.

3. Pasta with Pesto and Cherry Tomatoes:

- Cook your favorite pasta.
- Toss with fresh pesto sauce and halved cherry tomatoes.
- Top with grated Parmesan cheese.

4. Vegetarian Quesadillas:

- Fill whole wheat tortillas with black beans, corn, diced tomatoes, and cheese.
- Cook in a skillet until the tortillas are crispy and the cheese is melted.

5. Teriyaki Chicken Bowl:

- Sauté chicken strips in teriyaki sauce.
- Serve over quinoa or brown rice with steamed broccoli and sliced green onions.

6. Caprese Salad with Grilled Chicken:

- Grill chicken breasts and slice.
- Arrange on a plate with fresh mozzarella, cherry tomatoes, and basil leaves.
- Drizzle with balsamic glaze.

7. Sheet Pan Fajitas:

- Toss sliced bell peppers, onions, and chicken strips with fajita seasoning.
- Spread on a baking sheet and bake until the chicken is cooked and veggies are tender.
- Serve in tortillas with your favorite toppings.

8. Mushroom and Spinach Omelet:

- Whisk eggs and pour into a hot skillet.
- Add sautéed mushrooms and spinach.
- Fold the omelet and cook until the eggs are set.

9. Salmon and Asparagus Foil Packets:

- Place salmon filets and asparagus spears on a sheet of foil.
- Drizzle with olive oil, lemon juice, and season.

-   Seal the foil and bake until the salmon is flaky.

10. **Mango Chicken Lettuce Wraps:**

-   Cook diced chicken with mango chunks and a bit of soy sauce.
-   Spoon into lettuce leaves and garnish with chopped cilantro and lime.

12

TIPS FOR DINING OUT

Making DASH-Friendly Choices at Restaurants

When dining out while following the DASH (Dietary Approaches to Stop Hypertension) diet, here are some tips for making healthier choices:

1. **Start with Vegetables:**

   - Begin your meal with a salad or vegetable-based appetizer.
   - Opt for salads with a variety of colorful veggies, and choose a vinaigrette dressing on the side.

2. **Lean Protein Options:**

   - Choose lean protein sources such as grilled chicken, fish, or lean cuts of beef or pork.
   - Avoid fried or breaded protein options.

3. **Whole Grains:**

   - Opt for whole grain options when available, such as brown rice, quinoa, or whole wheat pasta.
   - Choose whole grain or multigrain bread over white bread.

4. **Limit Sodium:**

   - Ask for dishes to be prepared with less salt, and avoid adding extra salt at the table.
   - Be cautious with processed and cured meats, as they tend to be high in sodium.

5. **Mindful Sides:**

- Choose sides that include vegetables or whole grains.
- Opt for baked or roasted potatoes over fries.

6. **Control Portions:**

- Be mindful of portion sizes; consider sharing larger dishes or taking leftovers home.
- Ask for dressings and sauces on the side to control the amount you consume.

7. **Healthy Cooking Methods:**

- Look for menu items that are grilled, steamed, baked, or broiled.
- Avoid fried or deep-fried options.

8. **Hydration Choices:**

- Opt for water, herbal tea, or other non-caloric beverages instead of sugary drinks.
- Limit alcohol intake, if applicable, to moderate levels.

9. **Customize Your Order:**

- Don't hesitate to ask for modifications or substitutions to make the meal healthier.
- Choose olive oil or vinegar-based dressings instead of creamy ones.

10. **Dessert Moderation:**

- If you choose to have dessert, share it with others to control portion sizes.
- Look for fruit-based desserts or those with limited added sugars.

Navigating Buffets with a DASH-Friendly Approach

When facing a buffet while following the DASH (Dietary Approaches to Stop Hypertension) diet, consider these tips for making healthier choices:

1. **Survey the Buffet:**

   - Take a walk around the buffet to see all the available options before filling your plate.
   - Identify the healthier choices like salads, grilled proteins, and vegetable-based dishes.

2. **Start with Vegetables:**

   - Begin your buffet journey by filling a significant portion of your plate with a variety of colorful vegetables.
   - Opt for salads with leafy greens, tomatoes, cucumbers, and other fresh veggies.

3. **Choose Lean Proteins:**

   - Select lean protein sources such as grilled chicken, turkey, or fish.
   - Limit or avoid fried or breaded proteins.

4. **Mindful Carbohydrates:**

   - Choose whole grains when available, such as brown rice, quinoa, or whole wheat pasta.
   - Consider the proportion of carbohydrates on your plate, and aim for balance.

5. **Be Wary of Sauces and Dressings:**

- Request dressings and sauces on the side, allowing you to control the amount you use.
- Opt for vinaigrettes or olive oil-based dressings instead of creamy options.

6. Watch Portion Sizes:

- Use smaller plates to help control portion sizes.
- Focus on quality rather than quantity, savoring each bite.

7. Mind the Salt:

- Be cautious with overly salty dishes, and consider asking for dishes with reduced salt if possible.
- Avoid adding extra salt at the table.

8. Stay Hydrated:

- Drink water or other non-caloric beverages to stay hydrated.
- Limit sugary drinks and alcoholic beverages.

9. Savor Desserts Mindfully:

- If you choose to have dessert, opt for fruit-based options or those with limited added sugars.
- Keep portion sizes small, or consider sharing desserts.

10. Practice Moderation:

- Allow yourself to enjoy a variety of foods but in moderation.
- Listen to your body's hunger and fullness cues to avoid overeating.

Making DASH-Friendly Choices at Restaurants

When dining out on the DASH (Dietary Approaches to Stop Hypertension) diet, consider these tips for making healthier choices:

1. **Review the Menu in Advance:**

   - Check the restaurant's menu online before going to make informed choices and avoid feeling rushed.

2. **Choose Grilled or Baked Proteins:**

   - Opt for grilled, baked, or broiled proteins like chicken, fish, or lean cuts of beef. Avoid fried or breaded options.

3. **Load Up on Vegetables:**

   - Prioritize vegetable-based dishes. Look for salads, steamed or roasted veggies, and vegetable sides.

4. **Control Portion Sizes:**
   - Be mindful of portion sizes. Consider sharing an entree or packing leftovers to avoid overeating.

5. **Request Modifications
:**
   - Don't hesitate to ask for modifications. Request dressings, sauces, or condiments on the side to control portions.

6. **Choose Whole Grains:**

   - Opt for whole grain options when available. Choose whole wheat bread, brown rice, or quinoa.

7. **Limit Sodium:**

- Ask for dishes to be prepared with less salt. Avoid adding extra salt at the table. Be cautious with high-sodium menu items.

8. Be Wary of Hidden Sugars:

- Be mindful of added sugars. Choose beverages without added sugars, and be cautious with desserts.

9. Opt for Healthy Fats:

- Choose dishes with healthy fats such as olive oil or avocado. Limit saturated and trans fats.

10. Balance Your Plate:

- Aim for a balanced plate with a mix of lean proteins, vegetables, and whole grains. Create a well-rounded meal.

11. Consider Appetizers as Meals:

- Look at appetizers as potential meals. Sometimes they offer smaller portions and healthier options.

12. Choose Smart Side Dishes:

- Opt for side dishes that include vegetables, whole grains, or salads instead of fries or other fried options.

13. Be Mindful of Beverages:

- Choose water, herbal tea, or other non-caloric beverages instead of sugary drinks. Limit alcohol intake to moderate levels if applicable.

14. Ask for Nutritional Information:

- If available, ask for nutritional information. Some restaurants provide details about calorie content and nutritional values.

15. **Plan for Dessert Mindfully:**

- If you decide on dessert, consider sharing or choosing a fruit-based option with limited added sugars.

13

FAQs & TROUBLESHOOTING

Common Questions about the DASH Diet

1. What is the DASH Diet?

The DASH (Dietary Approaches to Stop Hypertension) diet is a dietary plan designed to help prevent and manage hypertension (high blood pressure). It emphasizes fruits, vegetables, whole grains, lean proteins, and low-fat dairy while limiting sodium and processed foods.

2. Is the DASH Diet Suitable for Weight Loss?

While the primary goal of the DASH diet is to lower blood pressure, many people find it effective for weight loss due to its emphasis on whole, nutrient-dense foods. It can be part of a healthy weight management plan.

3. Can I Eat Out on the DASH Diet?

Yes, you can eat out while following the DASH diet. Choose grilled proteins, salads, and vegetable-based dishes. Request dressings and sauces on the side to control portions, and be mindful of high-sodium options.

4. How Does the DASH Diet Impact Sodium Intake?

The DASH diet recommends limiting sodium intake to help lower blood pressure. It encourages choosing fresh, whole foods and avoiding processed and packaged foods high in sodium.

5. Can I Follow the DASH Diet if I Have Dietary Restrictions?
The DASH diet can be adapted to various dietary restrictions, such as vegetarian or gluten-free. It provides flexibility in food choices, making it suitable for different preferences and needs.

6. Is the DASH Diet Suitable for Everyone?

The DASH diet is generally suitable for most individuals. However, it's advisable to consult with a healthcare professional or registered dietitian before starting any new diet, especially for those with specific health conditions or dietary concerns.

7. How Does the DASH Diet Impact Cholesterol Levels?

The DASH diet's focus on whole foods, rich in fiber and healthy fats, can contribute to improved cholesterol levels. It emphasizes reducing saturated fat and increasing heart-healthy fats.

8. Can I Drink Alcohol on the DASH Diet?

Moderate alcohol consumption may be acceptable for some individuals following the DASH diet. However, it's important to limit alcoholic beverages and consider the impact on overall health and blood pressure.

9. Can I Snack on the DASH Diet?

Yes, snacking is allowed on the DASH diet. Choose healthy snacks like fresh fruit, vegetables with hummus, Greek yogurt, or a small handful of nuts. Be mindful of portion sizes.

10. Is the DASH Diet Sustainable Long-Term?

Many people find the DASH diet sustainable long-term because it encourages a balanced and varied intake of nutrient-dense foods. It can be adapted to individual preferences, making it a lifestyle rather than a short-term solution.

Overcoming Challenges on the DASH Diet

1. Sodium Reduction:

Challenge: Lowering sodium intake can be challenging, especially with processed and restaurant foods.
Solution: Choose fresh, whole foods, cook at home, and use herbs and spices for flavor. Gradually reduce added salt to allow taste buds to adjust.

2. Meal Preparation Time:

Challenge: Busy schedules may make it difficult to find time for meal preparation.

Solution: Plan and prep meals in advance, use time-saving kitchen tools, and explore quick and simple DASH-friendly recipes.

3. Dining Out:

Challenge: Limited DASH-friendly options at restaurants.
Solution: Check restaurant menus online beforehand, choose grilled or steamed options, and ask for modifications, such as dressing on the side.

4. Budget Constraints:

Challenge: Fresh, whole foods can sometimes be perceived as more expensive.
Solution: Buy in-season produce, choose frozen fruits and vegetables, and look for sales or discounts. Planning meals can also reduce food waste.

5. Social Events:

Challenge: Navigating social gatherings with different food options.
Solution: Bring a DASH-friendly dish to share, communicate dietary preferences, and focus on portion control while enjoying the company.

6. Vegetable Intake:

Challenge: Meeting the recommended vegetable servings daily.
Solution: Incorporate vegetables into every meal, try new recipes, and experiment with various cooking methods to enhance flavors.

7. Whole Grain Choices:

Challenge: Limited whole grain options in certain settings.
Solution: Choose whole grain varieties when available, such as brown rice, whole wheat bread, or quinoa. Substitute when possible.

8. Balancing Macronutrients:

Challenge: Finding the right balance of carbohydrates, proteins, and fats.
Solution: Use online resources to create balanced meals, consult with a registered dietitian, and experiment with portion sizes to find what works for you.

9. Adapting to Preferences:

Challenge: Adapting the DASH diet to personal preferences.
Solution: Explore various recipes, find DASH-friendly foods you enjoy, and customize the diet to suit your taste while maintaining nutritional balance.

10. Consistency:

Challenge: Maintaining consistency with the DASH diet over time.
Solution: Set realistic goals, celebrate small victories, and focus on the long-term benefits of a heart-healthy lifestyle. Incorporate variety to keep meals interesting.

14

CONCLUSION

Celebrating Your DASH Diet Journey

1. Milestone Reflection:

- Take a moment to reflect on your DASH diet journey. Celebrate milestones, whether it's sticking to the plan for a week, a month, or achieving a specific health goal.

2. Health Check-In:

- Schedule a health check-up to monitor any improvements in blood pressure, cholesterol levels, or overall well-being. Celebrate positive changes and use them as motivation.

3. Try New Recipes:

- Celebrate by trying out new DASH-friendly recipes. Experimenting with flavors and ingredients keeps the journey exciting and enjoyable.

4. Fitness Achievements:

- Acknowledge and celebrate any improvements in your fitness routine. Whether it's reaching a step goal, lifting more weight, or achieving a personal best, celebrate your physical accomplishments.

5. Mindful Eating Practices:

- Celebrate moments of mindful eating. Recognize when you make intentional and health-conscious food choices, savoring each bite and appreciating the nourishment.

6. Positive Habit Formation:

- Recognize the positive habits formed during your DASH diet journey. Celebrate the incorporation of more fruits, vegetables, and whole foods into your daily routine.

7. Share Success Stories:

- Share your DASH diet success stories with friends or family. Celebrate your achievements and inspire others to embrace a heart-healthy lifestyle.

8. Create a Visual Diary:

- Create a visual diary or vision board to track your DASH diet journey. Include inspirational quotes, images of favorite DASH-friendly meals, and reminders of your health goals.

9. Reward System:

- Establish a reward system for reaching milestones. Treat yourself to a non-food reward, such as a relaxing day, a new book, or an activity you enjoy.

10. Community Engagement:

- Join or create a community of individuals following the DASH diet. Celebrate achievements together, share tips, and provide support for one another.

11. Gratitude Practice:

- Cultivate gratitude for the positive changes in your life through the DASH diet. Celebrate the journey by acknowledging the impact on your overall well-being.

12. Self-Compassion:

- Practice self-compassion. Celebrate not only the successes but also acknowledge challenges overcome. Be kind to yourself during the journey.

Continuing a Heart-Healthy Lifestyle

1. Regular Health Check-ups:

- Schedule regular health check-ups to monitor blood pressure, cholesterol levels, and overall cardiovascular health. Stay informed about your progress and any adjustments needed.

2. Physical Activity Routine:

- Maintain a consistent physical activity routine. Aim for at least 150 minutes of moderate-intensity exercise per week, such as brisk walking, cycling, or swimming.

3. Diverse and Colorful Diet:

- Continue to enjoy a diverse and colorful diet rich in fruits, vegetables, whole grains, lean proteins, and low-fat dairy. Explore new recipes to keep meals exciting.

4. Hydration Habits:

- Stay hydrated by drinking plenty of water throughout the day. Limit sugary drinks and be mindful of alcohol intake.

5. Mindful Eating Practices:

- Practice mindful eating by savoring each bite, paying attention to hunger and fullness cues, and being present during meals.

6. Regular Sleep Patterns:

- Prioritize regular sleep patterns. Aim for 7-9 hours of quality sleep per night to support overall health and well-being.

7. Stress Management Techniques:

- Implement stress management techniques such as deep breathing, meditation, or yoga. Find activities that promote relaxation and balance in your life.

8. **Social Support:**

- Maintain a supportive network of friends and family. Share your heart-healthy journey with loved ones, and encourage each other to make health-conscious choices.

9. **Limit Added Sugars and Processed Foods:**

- Be mindful of added sugars and processed foods. Read labels, choose whole, minimally processed foods, and limit intake of high-sugar snacks and beverages.

10. **Regular Health Education:**

- Stay informed about heart health. Keep up with the latest health guidelines, research, and information to make informed decisions about your lifestyle.

11. **Set Realistic Goals:**

- Continue to set realistic and achievable goals. Whether it's maintaining a certain weight, increasing exercise intensity, or trying new heart-healthy recipes, establish goals that align with your lifestyle.

12. **Celebrate Achievements:**

- Celebrate ongoing achievements. Acknowledge both small and significant successes in your heart-healthy journey to stay motivated and positive.

13. **Adapt and Evolve:**

- Be flexible and willing to adapt your heart-healthy lifestyle as needed. Life circumstances may change, so adjust your routines and habits accordingly.

14. **Educate Others:**

- Share your heart-healthy knowledge with others. Encourage friends and family to adopt heart-healthy habits, creating a supportive environment for everyone.